An Atlas of Investigation and Management

HYPERTENSION

An Atlas of Investigation and Management

HYPERTENSION

Edward D Frohlich
Alton Ochsner Medical Foundation
New Orleans, USA

Hector O Ventura
Alton Ochsner Medical Foundation
New Orleans, USA

CLINICAL PUBLISHING
OXFORD

Clinical Publishing
an imprint of Atlas Medical Publishing Ltd
Oxford Centre for Innovation
Mill Street, Oxford OX2 0JX, UK

Tel: +44 1865 811116
Fax: +44 1865 251550
E mail: info@clinicalpublishing.co.uk
Web: www.clinicalpublishing.co.uk

Distributed in USA and Canada by:
Clinical Publishing
30 Amberwood Parkway
Ashland OH 44805 USA

tel: 800-247-6553 (toll free within U.S. and Canada)
fax: 419-281-6883
email: order@bookmasters.com

Distributed in UK and Rest of World by:
Marston Book Services Ltd
PO Box 269
Abingdon
Oxon OX14 4YN UK

tel: +44 1235 465500
fax: +44 1235 465555
e mail: trade.orders@marston.co.uk

First published 2009

A catalogue record for this book is available from the British Library

ISBN-13 978 1 904392 15 6
ISBN-10 1 904392 15 6
ISBN e-book 978 1 84692 524 5

Project managed by Prepress Projects Ltd, Perth, UK
Typeset by Initial Typesetting Services, Edinburgh, UK
Printed by T G Hostench, s.a.

Contents

Preface and a brief apologia

In a textbook of this nature, it is in order to provide the prospective reader and potential reviewer with a brief overview of the goals, limits and editorial guidelines that we set for ourselves in preparing the material for this atlas. In the Introduction we provide some personal remarks related to our agreement to organize and present our repertoire of visual material, but, perhaps, a few words might be in order here to explain our selection.

First, a number of friends and colleagues encouraged us to publish the material for many of our lectures over the years. Our publisher further supported these comments although he raised the concern that some material and references might seem to be dated. We agreed and exerted particular effort to select only that pictorial and diagrammatic material which we strongly believed was currently pertinent for presentation and for pedagogic purposes.

Another concern (as a past Editor-in-Chief of two major journals and the author of several textbooks and many papers) was related to our selection of reference material. The purpose of this text was to present neither a literature review nor a current state of the art. We therefore chose to provide 'suggested reading' so that the reader can consult in the peer-reviewed literature the primary references for the clinical and experimental material we use to support our pictorial, tabular and diagrammatic material.

With these comments, we sincerely hope that the atlas material, the accompanying discussion and suggested reading are of value to the reader. We hope that this book will be of value to readers who are clinicians and students of hypertension and who are interested in the pathophysiology of hypertensive disease.

Abbreviations

ACE	angiotensin-converting enzyme
ACEI	angiotensin-converting enzyme inhibitor
ARB	angiotensin receptor blocker
AT	angiotensinogen
AV	arteriolar–venular
BB	beta blocker
CBC	complete blood count
CCB	calcium channel blocker
CHD	coronary heart disease
CHF	congestive heart failure
COPD	chronic obstructive pulmonary disease
CPV	cardiopulmonary volume
DBP	diastolic blood pressure
ECG	electrocardiogram
ERBF	estimated renal blood flow
ESRD	end-stage renal disease
FF	filtration fraction
GFR	glomerular filtration rate
HCTZ	hydrochlorothiazide
HCVD	hypertensive cardiovascular disease
HHD	hypertensive heart disease
IP3	inositol triphosphate
ISA	intrinsic sympathomimetic activity
IVU	intravenous urography
LV	left ventricle
LVH	left ventricular hypertrophy
LVS	left ventricular strain
MAP	mean arterial pressure
MI	myocardial infarction
L-NAME	nitro-L-arginine methyl ester hydrochloride
NSAID	non-steroidal anti-inflammatory drug
PKD	polycystic kidney disease
PRA	plasma renin activity
PSA	prostate-specific antigen
PV	plasma volume
PWT	pulmonary wall thickness
RA	renal afferent
RE	renal efferent
RHD	rheumatic heart disease
SHR	spontaneously hypertensive rat
SBP	systolic blood pressure
SNFF	single-nephron filtration fraction
SNGFR	single-nephron glomerular filtration rate
SNPF	single-nephron plasma flow
SMA	smooth muscle actin
TPR	total peripheral resistance
TSH	thyroid-stimulating hormone
UPE	urinary protein excretion
WKY	Wistar–Kyoto rat

Dedication

We dedicate this textbook to our wives, Sherry Frohlich and Laurie Ventura, and to our children, who share with us the very honest and warm thirst for knowledge, whether in the medical or in other academic environments. It is this understanding of the need to impart one's personal or professional knowledge and experience which provides an added dimension to nurture family as well as our professional colleagues. This is the long-standing commitment of the well-rounded physician, and it is the obligation of all teachers and professionals to impart a better life to man within our professional careers.

Introduction

Producing an atlas on hypertension was not at the forefront of my thinking until I was approached by Jonathan Gregory, commissioning editor at Clinical Publishing, who was interested in publishing such a textbook. Indeed, in recent years, I have questioned the importance of hypertension as a discipline. Institutions such as mine no longer maintain a separate hospital service for admitting patients with the diagnosis of hypertension; and the numbers of patients with primary problems relating to hypertension have diminished considerably. This is in striking contrast to the early days of my academic career, when a large majority of hospitalized patients were admitted with hypertensive emergencies or hypertension associated with myocardial infarction, congestive heart failure, angina pectoris, stroke or renal involvement. Today, a patient with hypertension who is hospitalized because of myocardial infarction, acute coronary syndrome or renal failure is immediately sent to a specialized unit. Yes, we have certainly come a long way over the past five decades.

On the other hand, the number of patients with hypertension continues to increase all over the world. Clearly, this is partly the result of what I have termed the 'numbers game' of disease. That is to say, the limits of normal – whether of blood pressure, blood sugar concentration or body weight – continue to converge, and so the number of potential patients with hypertension or diabetes mellitus or obesity continues to rise. And as a consequence, the increasing attention demanded by these diseases falls on the shoulders of the primary care physician, and with this responsibility comes a greater need for a clear understanding of the pathophysiology of these diseases and their management. Related to the increased attention these diseases receive, and the increase in the number of such patients seen in any physician's day-to-day practice, are remarkable innovations in diagnosis and management. And so the subject arose of yet another textbook about hypertension. I was won over by the need to confine the text to just these subjects: classification of the disease; a clear insight into the pathophysiology and initial evaluation of the hypertensive patient; an elucidation of the mechanisms of action of the varied modes of therapy including non-drug as well as pharmacological entities; and my personal overview and investigative and clinical experience with two vital areas, the heart and kidney in hypertension.

Most national and international guidelines present a straightforward concept for the evaluation and treatment of patients with hypertension; and they presently suggest a clear-cut course of action with respect to treatment unless there are complicating considerations. For the most part, we agree with this presentation; but, of course, as is the case with most consultants, consideration must be focused on the patient in whom complicating factors suggest specific problems. To my way of thinking, the major areas that require more specific attention relate to the hypertensive patient with cardiac or renal involvement. Indeed, cardiac and renal failure continue to increase in frequency despite the reduction in deaths from stroke or coronary heart disease and the fact that hypertensive emergencies are today rather rare. Patients with hypertension who are hospitalized with myocardial infarction or with end-stage renal disease, as well as patients with an acute stroke, require very specialized hospital services. And so we are left with the need to consider in detail the heart in hypertension and the kidney in hypertension. Both deserve very specific discussions in a textbook for the primary care physician or internist, cardiologist or nephrologist, all of whom deal with a large number of such patients who are not covered adequately by current clinical guidelines. Moreover, over the past few years I have on several occasions been invited to present my thoughts on this matter to such physicians, and so I was convinced that now might be an appropriate time to share my personal thoughts in an 'atlas' format. It became apparent to me that in such a book I would be able to impart not only my personal clinical experience, but also the ongoing work in my laboratories, which focuses primarily on the heart and kidney. At this point in my thinking about the subject, I discussed the merits of the task with my long-time friend and colleague, Hector Ventura. Hector convinced me of the potential 'need' for such an undertaking, and when he 'volunteered' to assist me I readily agreed. Thus, the concept and the format for this atlas of hypertension developed and we thereupon began this job.

Not infrequently, we are invited to write a book review. Often, one of the major pitfalls for an author is to clearly identify what the book is trying to achieve; and so we were very careful to ensure that we express our thinking clearly. We did not want to write a textbook that deals with the hypertensive patient who presents with problems that constitute an emergency or those who require hospitalization in a special care unit. Nor did we want to discuss the patient whose demographic characteristics are such that specific chapters need be dedicated to a discussion of the role of the patient's age, race or gender, or the patient who suffers from a new popular syndrome. In the final analysis, when the physician is confronted by a particular patient, the relationship is one-on-one, and the decision about diagnosis and therapy for that person is very specific and unique for that clinical situation.

Thus, we accepted Jonathan Gregory's invitation and presented to him our revised thinking. We proposed a textbook that would present our personal opinions about hypertensive disease and its cardiac and renal complications as it relates to everyday pathophysiological assessment and about the choice of therapy not only for the relatively uncomplicated patient but also for the frequently encountered patient with complications affecting the heart and kidneys. This material would, we believe, best be presented as tables or figures that would hopefully clarify our thinking on patient management as suggested by our clinical as well as laboratory experience.

To complete our task we want to express our appreciation to Jonathan Gregory for stimulating our thinking about how to present the very common problem of hypertension in the practice setting. We also want to express our warm and heartfelt appreciation to our wives and children, first and foremost, for their abiding understanding of our need to spend more time away from home and family in order to meet yet another deeply personal commitment. It is to them, our dear families, that we dedicate this endeavour. In addition, we want to express our appreciation to our office staff (Lillian Buffa, Caramia Fairchild and Pamella Tadesco), whose continuous support of our daily professional activities permitted us to pursue yet another job.

It would be totally remiss of me not to mention a few stumbling blocks that I encountered along the way during the preparation of this book: the sudden striking of Hurricanes Katrina and Rita; the associated flooding and loss of my home and long-to-be remembered library (including 'saved' copies of completed chapters on hard drives and disks), records and recollections; an enforced evacuation from New Orleans to our daughter's home in Chicago; and conversation and support from my son in New Jersey whereby personal refocusing was made possible. And, finally, I want to express my (our) appreciation to our colleagues and institution, who continue to provide the ambience and culture required to pursue an academic dimension to the overall healthcare effort (especially in the past difficult times).

Edward D. Frohlich, MD
New Orleans, LA
May 2008

Chapter 1

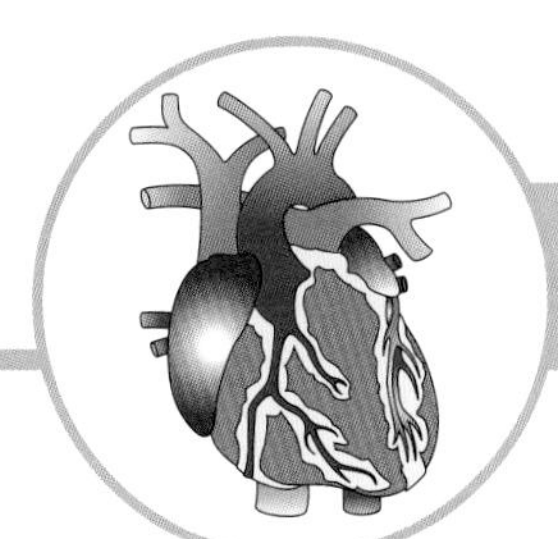

Pathophysiology: disease mechanisms

Introduction

Systemic arterial hypertension is one of the most common cardiovascular diseases of industrialized populations. It affects approximately 20% of adults in these societies, and a much higher proportion in certain demographic groups (e.g. blacks, the elderly). The disease is the major treatable risk factor underlying coronary heart disease (*Table 1.1*), and exacerbates and accelerates the atherosclerotic process. Moreover, hypertension is a key determinant risk for premature cardiovascular morbidity and mortality end-points (*Table 1.2*). It is, therefore, necessary to understand the nature of the disease pathophysiologically; by doing so, it is then possible to conceive, develop, and select. This, then, is the mission of this atlas.

Table 1.1 Risk factors underlying coronary heart disease

Not treatable
- Advancing age
- Male gender
- Black race
- Positive family history

Treatable
- Hypertension
- Hyperlipidaemia
- Tobacco consumption
- Obesity
- Diabetes mellitus

Unresolved (as to whether treatment reverses risk)
- Left ventricular hypertrophy
- Hyperinsulinism
- Hyperuricaemia
- Indices of inflammation (e.g. C-reactive protein)

Table 1.2 Complications and end-points promoted by hypertension that result in premature cardiovascular morbidity and mortality

Brain
- Haemorrhagic stroke
- Thrombotic stroke
- Embolic stroke

Heart
- Angina pectoris involving coronary arterioles
- Occlusive epicardial coronary arterial diseases
- Congestive heart failure
- Left ventricular diastolic dysfunction

Kidney
- Renal arterial disease
- End-stage renal disease
- Embolic renal disease
- Exacerbation of diabetic renal disease

Other hypertensive emergencies
- Dissecting aortic aneurysm
- Accelerated and malignant hypertension
- Crisis from phaeochromocytoma
- Eclampsia
- Other pressor emergencies

The mosaic

It was approximately 60 years ago that Irvine H. Page described his concept of the mosaic of hypertension (see Further reading). Inherent in his thesis was the belief that hypertension is multifactorial in causation. This is because all of the mechanisms that serve to control arterial pressure in normal individuals as well as in those patients with hypertensive disease relate to each other in a kaleidoscopic fashion, each with the others. Thus, all mechanisms are critical for maintaining homeostasis, physiologically or pathophysiologically (**1.1A, B**).

The factors depicted in Page's mosaic clearly are not all-inclusive but serve to satisfy the underlying model suggesting that many (if not most) diseases are multifactorial in causation. In the case of hypertension, the fundamental driving physiological purpose is to maintain normal tissue perfusion. In hypertension, this is accomplished at the expense of an increased vascular resistance and, hence, the elevated arterial pressure which is the primary clinical characteristic of hypertensive disease.

Altered haemodynamics

To understand the pathophysiological alterations associated with the systemic arterial hypertensive diseases, there must first be a clear-cut understanding of the haemodynamic alterations associated with a persistent elevation of arterial pressure. By definition, hypertension is a haemodynamic disorder in which the elevated arterial pressure may be associated with an increased cardiac output and/or total peripheral resistance (**1.2**).

In most patients with essential hypertension, the elevated arterial pressure is associated with an increased total peripheral resistance. In some patients, however, an elevated cardiac output may also participate. The relationship between arterial pressure, cardiac output, and total peripheral resistance is discussed more extensively in subsequent chapters. However, when one considers the magnitude of the elevated pressure, changes in blood viscosity do not have major importance. Nevertheless, intravascular rheological changes may alter local tissue blood flow dynamics in the major target organs. Thus, it is possible that some degree of increased viscosity promotes changes in blood rheological characteristics which could

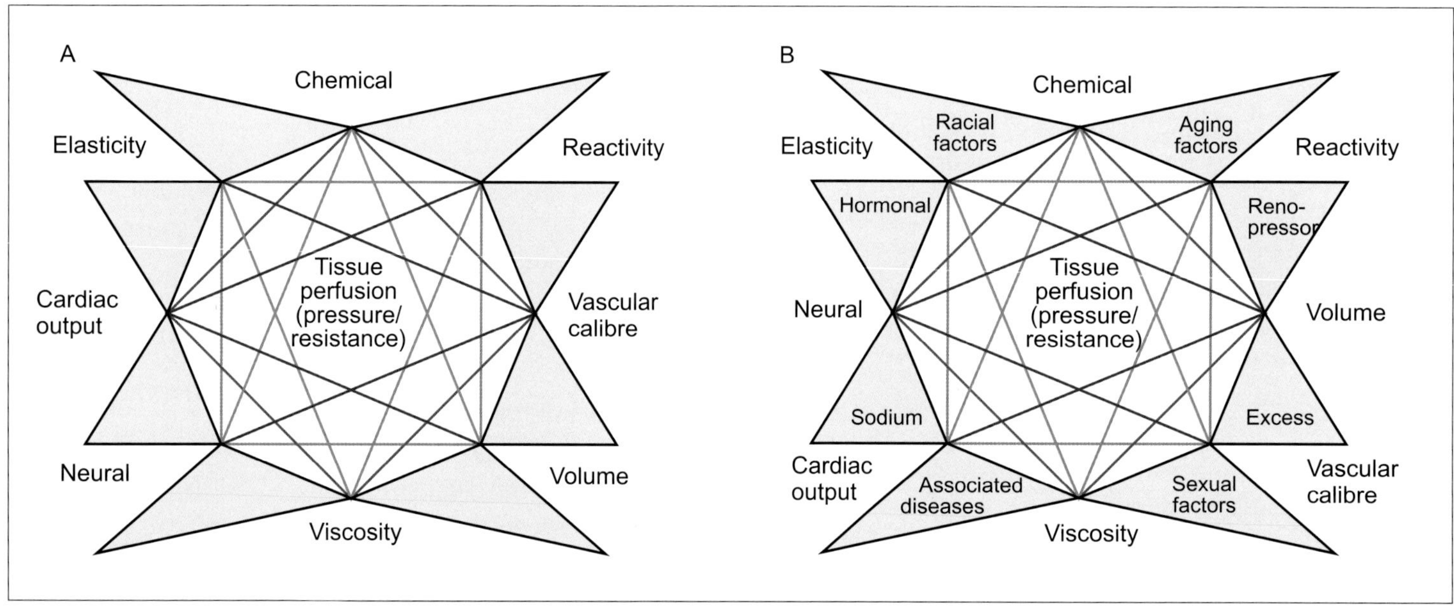

1.1 Page's mosaic theory of hypertension. **A**: the original theory; **B**: including additional factors as modified by the author. Each of these (and other) factors interrelate with one another in order to maintain normal tissue perfusion in response to an increasing vascular resistance and at the expense of the abnormally elevated arterial pressure. (Modified from Frohlich ED: Clinical classifications of hypertensive diseases. In: *Atherosclerosis and Coronary Artery Disease*. V Fuster, R Ross, E Topol (eds.). Lippincott-Raven, Philadelphia, 1996.)

exacerbate the haemodynamic alterations in the coronary, renal, and brain circulations.

For the most part, however, the increased total peripheral resistance (or, in organ circulations, their corresponding vascular resistances) is the established haemodynamic hallmark of the hypertension and is more or less uniformly distributed throughout the various organ circulations. The mechanism responsible for this resistance increase is an augmented vascular smooth muscle tone, primarily in the precapillary arterioles, and accounts for the state of increased arteriolar tone (i.e. arteriolar constriction) that is implicit in the multifactorial nature of the disease (*Table 1.3*).

Table 1.3 Active and passive mechanisms that alter vascular resistance

I. Constriction	II. Dilatation
Active • Adrenergic stimulation (i.e. increased neural input or increased vascular responsiveness to normal neural input) • Catecholamines: norepinephrine (noradrenaline), epinephrine (adrenaline), dopamine • Renopressor: angiotensin II • Cations: Ca^{2+}, K^+ (high concentration) • Other humoral substances: vasopressin, serotonin, certain endothelins, certain prostaglandins *Passive* • Oedema: extravascular compression • Vessel wall waterlogging • Increased blood or plasma viscosity • Obstruction (proximal): thrombosis, embolus, rarefaction • Hyposmolarity • Temperature: cold	*Active* • Acetylcholine • Nitric oxide • Kinins: bradykinin, kallidin • Prostaglandins (some) • Catecholamines: low-dose epinephrine (adrenaline), dopamine • Histamines • Peptides (atrial natriuretic peptide, insulin, secretin, vasoactive intestinal polypeptide, parathormone, calcitonin gene-related peptide, substance P, endorphins, enkephalins) • Renal medullary phospholipid substance (medullin) • Cations: K^+ (low concentration), Mg^{2+} • Vasoactive metabolites: adenosine, Krebs intermediate metabolites, acetate *Passive* • Reduced blood or plasma viscosity • Increased plasma tonicity • Hyperosmolarity • Temperature: heat

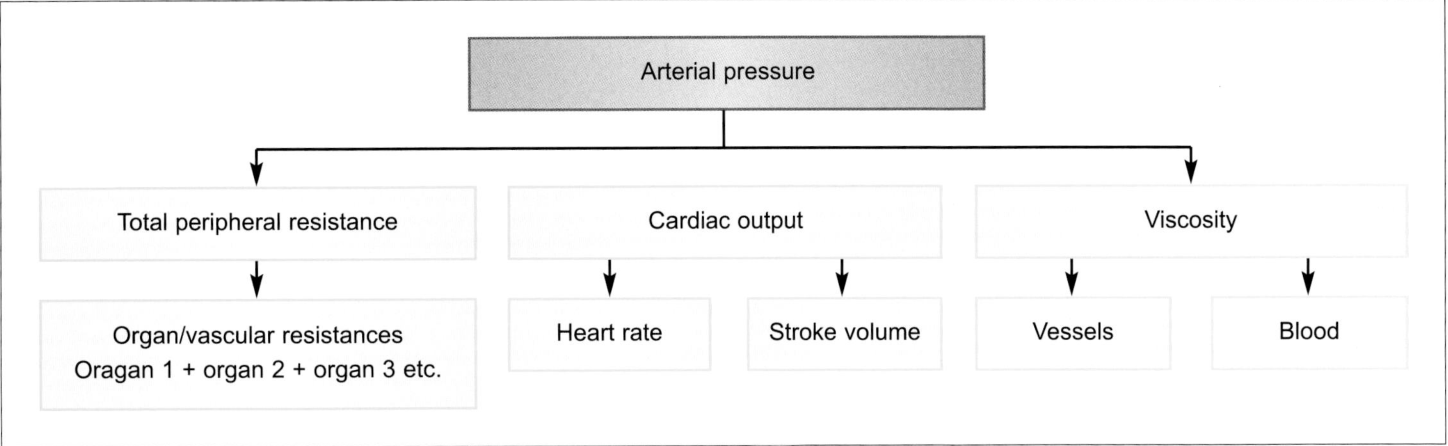

1.2 The haemodynamic concept inherent in hypertension.

This book emphasizes those mechanisms that have been related to essential hypertension, since this primary form of hypertension occurs in approximately 95% of all patients with systemic arterial hypertension. Moreover, this pathophysiological discussion is also relevant to other (i.e. secondary) clinical forms of hypertension. Consideration of the pertinent underlying pressor mechanisms in those secondary forms of hypertension provides a basis for a more comprehensive insight into the overall mechanisms that could participate in patients with essential hypertension (*Table 1.4*).

Table 1.4 Classification of the various forms of systemic arterial hypertension

Primary (essential) hypertension (hypertension of undetermined cause)
- Borderline (labile) or 'high normal' hypertension or prehypertension (essential hypertension)
- Essential hypertension: systolic pressures >139 mmHg and diastolic pressures >89 mmHg
- Isolated systolic hypertension: systolic pressures >139 mmHg with diastolic pressures <89 mmHg

Secondary hypertension
- Aortic coarctation

Central nervous system diseases
- Increased spinal fluid pressure
- Tumours
- Diencephalic syndrome

Renal arterial disease (renovascular hypertension)
- Non-atherosclerotic (fibrosing): intimal fibroplasia, medial fibroplasia, fibromuscular hyperplasia, subadventitial fibroplasia
- Atherosclerotic
- Aneurysm(s) of renal artery
- Embolic
- Extravascular compression (of renal artery): tumour, fibrosis
- Perinephric hull (Page kidney)
- Exacerbation of diabetic renal disease

Renal parenchymal disease
- Chronic pyelonephritis
- Acute glomerulonephritis
- Chronic glomerulonephritis
- Polycystic renal disease
- Diabetic nephropathy
- Others: amyloidosis, ureteral obstruction

Hormonal disease
- Thyroid
- Hyperthyroidism
- Hypothyroidism
- Hashimoto's thyroiditis

Adrenal cortical hypertension
- Cushing's disease or Cushing's syndrome
- Primary hyperaldosteronism
- Bilateral hyperplasia
- Adrenal enzymatic deficiencies

Adrenal medullary hypertension (i.e. phaeochromocytoma)

Other endocrine
- Ectopic production of hormones (tumours)
- Growth hormone excess (e.g. acromegaly, gigantism)
- Hypercalcaemic diseases (e.g. hyperparathyroidism, milk-alkali syndrome, hypervitaminosis D, metastatic bone disease, idiopathic hypercalcaemia)
- Oral contraceptive-exacerbated hypertension

Drugs, chemicals, and foods
- Excessive alcohol intake
- Excessive dietary sodium intake
- Exogenously administered adrenal steroids
- Birth control pills
- Adrenal steroids for asthma, malignancies, anabolic steroids
- Liquorice excess (imported primarily from the Netherlands not synthetic in USA, UK)
- Cold preparations: phenylpropanolamine, nasal decongestants
- Snuff and tobacco
- Street drugs (e.g. cocaine)

Complications from specific therapies
- Antidepressant therapy (tricyclic antidepressants, MAO inhibitors)
- Chronic steroid administration
- Cyclosporine (transplantation and certain disease immunosuppressive therapy)
- Beta-adrenergic receptor agonists (e.g. for asthma)
- Radiation nephritis and arthritis
- Lithotripsy therapy for renal calculi

MAO, monoamine oxidase.

Arteriolar constriction

Arteriolar (and, for that matter, venular) smooth muscle tone is increased in hypertension, although all of the mechanism(s) responsible are not entirely known. No doubt, this relates to the many pressor and depressor factors that normally participate in regulating vessel tone and calibre and, hence, arterial pressure (*Table 1.3*). It follows that these factors also participate in the increased vascular resistance in most patients with essential hypertension. Lessons concerning regulation of increased vascular resistance have been learned from the variety of secondary forms of hypertension in which specific pressor and depressor mechanisms are involved (*Table 1.4*).

It is likely that the increased vascular resistance in most patients with essential hypertension may be mediated through more than one pressor mechanism. Some of these mechanisms are predetermined by inborn genetic factors, since it has become increasingly apparent that the pathophysiological alterations in essential hypertension are polygenetic in origin. Furthermore, many of the pressor and depressor mechanisms that seem to be operative have been well documented to increase actively vascular smooth muscle tone. Many new mechanisms are elucidated with each passing year. Thus, vascular smooth muscle tone is abnormally increased as a result of one or more of those factors that participate in the underlying disease process and are then expressed in the clinical manifestations of that patient's disease. As a consequence of the increased total peripheral resistance, arterial pressure rises in order to maintain tissue perfusion; this occurs at the expense of the vascular and cardiac systems, and the specific indices of organ damage and functional impairment that secondarily result.

As suggested in *Tables 1.2* and *1.3*, the increased tone of the arteriolar or venular smooth muscle occurs no matter what mechanism(s) participate. Thus, for example, the vascular myocyte is constricted by enhanced adrenergic input or elevated circulating levels of catecholamines; alterations in circulating or local autocrine/paracrine effects of humoral substances; local or systemic participation of vasoactive peptides (e.g. angiotensin II, endothelin); ions; and growth factors. Alternatively, increased vascular resistance may also be produced by reduced local or systemic amounts of vasodilating agents, local vasoactive peptides or ions, and vasoactive metabolites (*Table 1.3*). Whatever the myocytic stimulus, there is a resultant rise in cytoplasmic free calcium ions from their resting state that results in enhanced phosphorylation of myosin light chains. This increased calcium ionic milieu may be achieved either through an inflow of calcium ions through calcium- or other receptor-activated membrane channels or by a release of calcium ions from intracellular organelles, although calcium may be released from the mitochondria or from binding with protein substrates through secondarily activated biochemical processes. The net increase in intracytoplasmic calcium ion concentration promotes the formation of inositol triphosphate (IP3) and diacylglycerol. IP3 serves as the second messenger, mediating the calcium ion release and the resulting mechanical coupling that permits an enhanced state of contractility of vascular smooth muscle.

Arteriolar structure

Another factor participating in the increased vascular resistance of hypertension is an increased wall-to-lumen ratio of the arteries and arterioles. This structural alteration in hypertension serves to amplify the arteriolar responsiveness to constrictor stimuli that maintains the hypertensive disease process. Recent investigations have suggested that the haemodynamic stress of vessel stretch may be an important additional mechanism responsible for the vessel wall thickening, or even of myocytic hypertrophy of the left ventricle. Several reports have indicated that upon stretch of the ventricular or arteriolar (e.g. renal, coronary) myocyte, one or more of a vast array of 'early genes' or proto-oncogenes participate in initiating DNA-directed myocytic and collagen (and likely other) growth. Some of these growth factors are themselves vasoconstrictors (e.g. angiotensin II, norepinephrine [noradrenaline], endothelin), and they may even be generated within the arteriolar or ventricular endothelium or wall itself. Intriguingly, they may also participate in the separate but related process of atherogenesis. Hence, this may explain the close relationship of these two common and comorbid diseases (i.e. hypertensive vascular disease and atherosclerosis).

Pre- and postcapillary constriction

For the most part, all patients with hypertension have an increased arterial pressure that is associated with an increased contractile state of vascular smooth muscle in both the arterioles and venules. The movement of plasma or interstitial fluid across the capillaries follows Starling mechanics, and depends upon the hydrostatic and colloid osmotic pressures in the intravascular and interstitial compartments, respectively (**1.3**). Additionally, the wall-to-lumen ratio of the arterioles, which is increased in hypertension, further increases vascular resistance and arterial pressure (i.e. the Folköwian hypothesis). The increased tone of the smooth muscle in the arteriolar wall is responsible for the increased arteriolar constriction. As a result of the constriction and, consequently, the increased total peripheral resistance and arterial pressure, left ventricular afterload increases *pari passu*, providing the major haemodynamic determinant for the structural ventricular adaptation of left ventricular hypertrophy and the associated events of hypertensive heart disease. These precapillary changes are associated with generalized constriction of the postcapillary venules, which reduces total body venous capacity. The simultaneous events of arteriolar and venular constriction relate to several pathophysiological phenomena and consequences of hypertensive disease (**1.4**).

Venoconstriction

The reduced venous capacity resulting from postcapillary venular constriction diminishes the overall venular capacity of the peripheral circulation. As a result, the circulating intravascular volume is redistributed from the periphery to the central circulation to increase venous return to the heart (i.e. cardiopulmonary volume) and, hence, cardiac output (**1.4**). This intravascular volume redistribution phenomenon has been demonstrated clinically in patients with essential hypertension as well as in naturally occurring or other experimental forms of hypertension. Thus, early in the development of hypertension, systemic venoconstriction may not be associated with intravascular volume contraction (**1.4**). However, as arteriolar and venular constriction progresses, capillary hydrostatic pressure increases and circulating intravascular volume diminishes. This is probably the consequence of two factors: movement of plasma from the circulation into the extravascular compartment and renal excretion of some of the circulating volume as arterial pressure increases (i.e. the Guytonian phenomenon of pressure natriuresis). The intravascular (i.e. plasma) volume contraction results in other recognizable factors (*Table 1.5*). Thus, as diastolic and mean arterial pressures or total peripheral resistance increase in hypertensive patients with essential hypertension or with renal arterial disease, plasma volume contracts (**1.5A**, **B**, **C**) and renal parenchymal disease.

In contrast, patients with parenchymal disease of the kidney demonstrate an increased plasma volume as diastolic pressure increases (**1.6**) due to renal mechanisms subserving volume expansion.

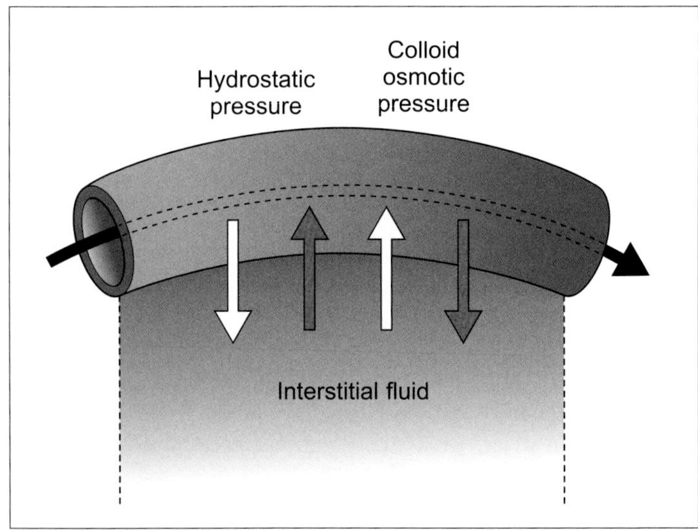

1.3. The four pressure determinants of transcapillary fluid migration elucidated by Starling.

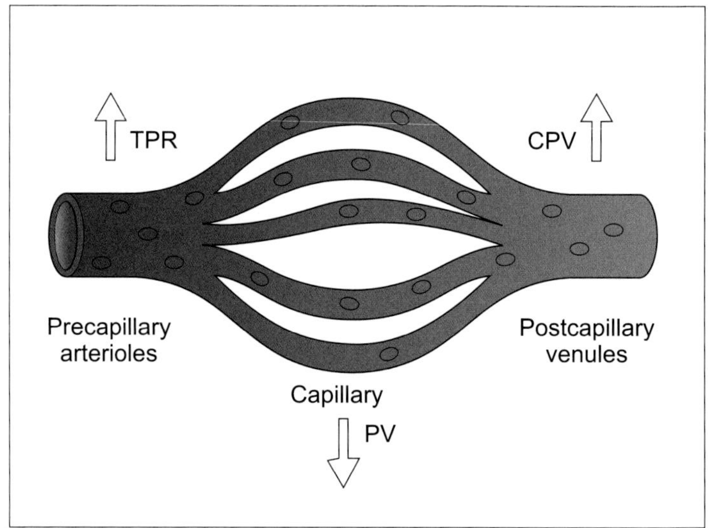

1.4. The role of pre- and postcapillary tone in regulating plasma volume. TPR, total peripheral resistance; PV, plasma volume; CPV, cardiopulmonary volume.

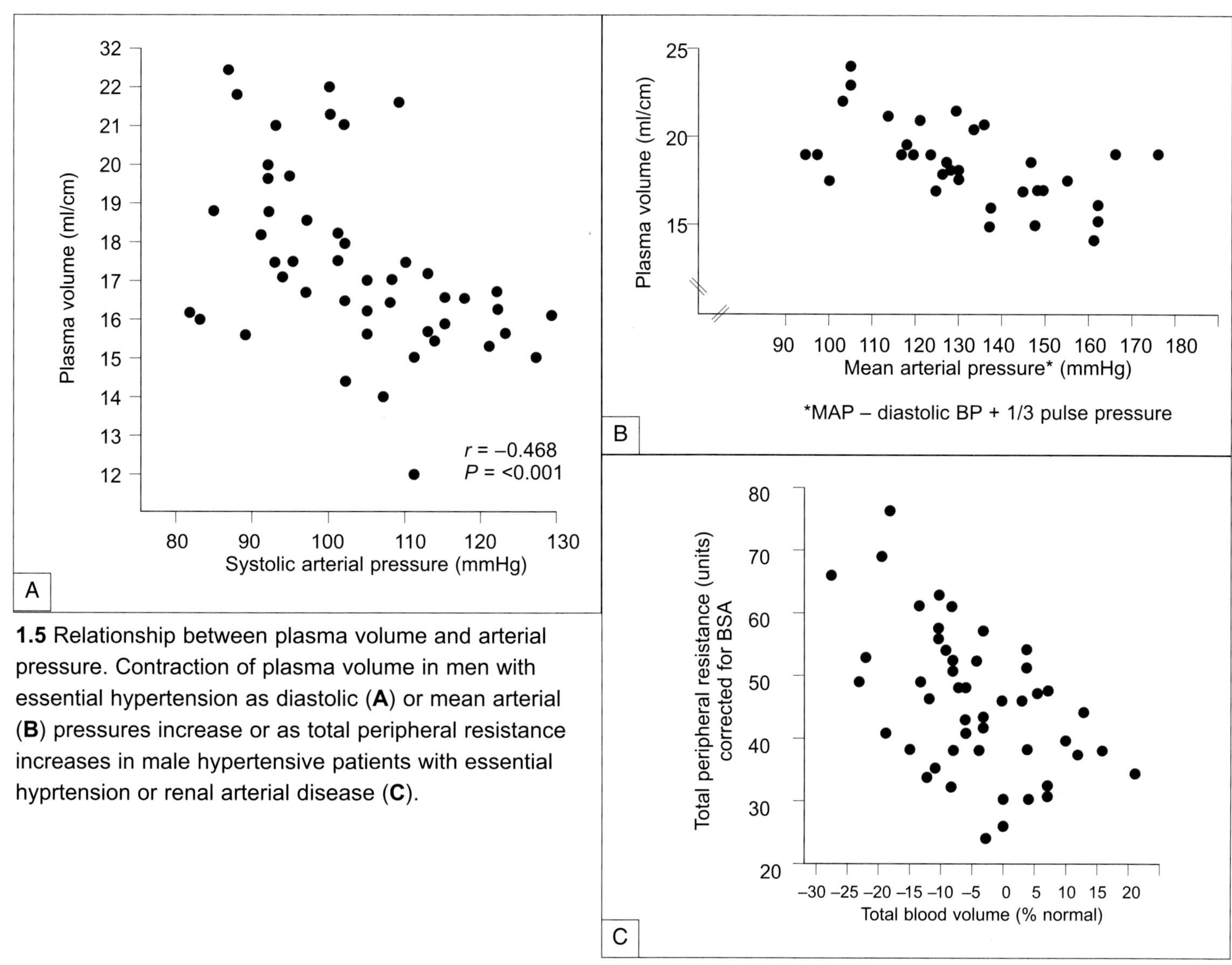

1.5 Relationship between plasma volume and arterial pressure. Contraction of plasma volume in men with essential hypertension as diastolic (**A**) or mean arterial (**B**) pressures increase or as total peripheral resistance increases in male hypertensive patients with essential hyprtension or renal arterial disease (**C**).

Table 1.5 Clinically recognizable correlates of contracted intravascular (plasma) volume

- Elevated haemoglobin concentration and haematocrit
- Increased plasma protein concentration (e.g. albumin, fibrinogen)
- Increased blood (and plasma) viscosity
- Hyperuricaemia

High haematocrit and haemoglobin

The higher haematocrit and haemoglobin levels in essential hypertension explain the clinical term 'reactive' or 'relative' polycythaemia. This entity is frequently detected in patients with essential hypertension and was first described by Gaisböck at the turn of the twentieth century. Unlike polycythaemia rubra vera, there is neither a leucocytosis or thrombocytosis, nor is there associated splenomegaly. The elevated haemoglobin and haematocrit in Gaisböck syndrome is classically described in the 'ruddy' patient with essential hypertension with contracted plasma volume. This relative increase in red cell mass with a reduced plasma volume has been measured in a large number of patients with essential hypertension. In contrast, some patients have a volume-dependent essential hypertension in whom the magnitude of plasma volume is directly related to the height of arterial pressure (*Table 1.6*).

This, then, provides an explanation why those patients with essential hypertension have plasma volume contraction may lose effective control of arterial pressure when they are treated only with an adrenergic inhibitor or a direct acting, smooth muscle relaxing vasodilators (e.g. sodium nitroprusside in the intensive care situation). Thus, plasma volume expands as pressure is reduced with treatment and, under these conditions, blood pressure control can then be restored with diuretic administration. Indeed, this explains the phenomenon of 'pseudotolerance' (**1.6**).

Table 1.6 Forms of hypertension associated with alterations of intravascular (plasma) volume

Contracted plasma volume

- Increasing severity of essential hypertension
- 'High-renin' essential hypertension
- Renal arterial disease
- Phaeochromocytoma

Expanded plasma volume

- Volume-dependent essential hypertension
  - – Low plasma renin activity
  - – Hypertension in black patients
- Steroid-dependent hypertension
  - – Primary hyperaldosteronism
  - – Cushing's disease or syndrome
- Renal parenchymal disease (including end-stage renal disease)
- Left ventricular failure
- Patients with prior contracted plasma volume treated with smooth muscle vasodilators and alpha-adrenergic receptor blocking agents

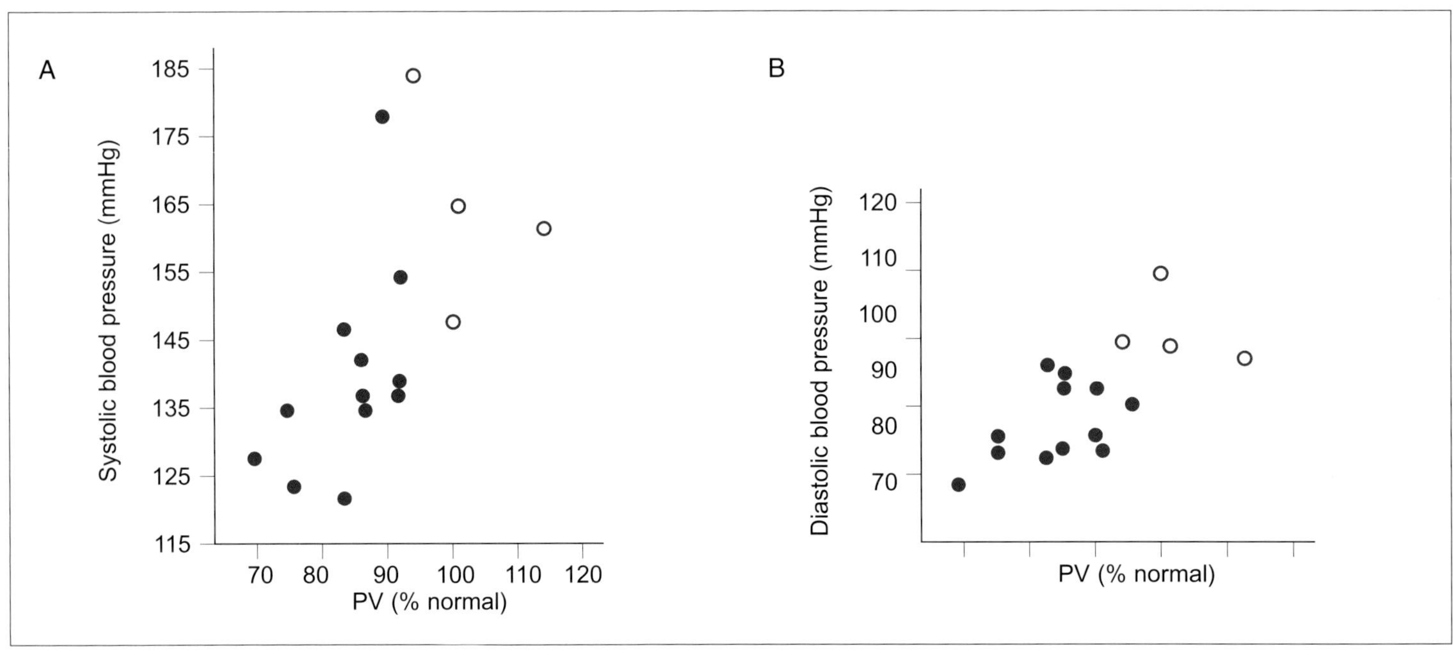

1.6 Expansion of plasma volume in patients with essential hypertension as systolic and diastolic pressures increase when adrenergic inhibitors or direct-acting smooth muscle relax vasodilators are used.

Oedema

A second clinical example of coincident pre- and postcapillary vasoconstriction may be demonstrated in those patients with severe hypertensive retinopathy. It provides an explanation for the transudation of protein through the retinal capillary bed in patients with accelerated hypertension as well as those with papilloedema associated with malignant hypertension (see Chapter 2). A third example relates to development of oedema in patients receiving calcium antagonists. This oedema is the consequence not of renal-mediated fluid retention but, rather, of the potent drug-induced precapillary arteriolar dilatation associated with reflex postcapillary constriction. This is particularly experienced with prolonged standing or when seated for a long time with the legs dependent.

High cardiac output hypertension

A fourth example of the phenomenon of pre- and post-capillary constriction provides, in part, a pathophysiological explanation for the increased cardiac output and hyper-dynamic circulation observed during development of essential hypertension. Thus, early in the elaboration of hypertension (i.e. patients with borderline or 'labile' hypertension), when blood pressure is elevated only at times but is normal at other times, cardiac output is increased. This increased output is related to the translocation of the circulating intravascular volume from the periphery to the central circulation as a result of the postcapillary (i.e. venular) constriction. Although the total peripheral resistance at this stage is said to be 'normal', it has been suggested that it is 'inappropriately so', since, should cardiac output become elevated to the same extent in normotensive individuals, their total peripheral resistance would be slightly reduced. With progression of the hypertensive vascular disease and, as the pre- and postcapillary vasoconstriction increase further, the intravascular (i.e. plasma) volume progressively contracts as described above. This contraction in circulating intravascular volume proportionally diminishes the cardiopulmonary volume, decreases right atrial venous return and, thus, the cardiac output is reduced to a more normal level than the output observed earlier in the disease.

Nephrosclerosis

A fifth example, which has more recently become appreciated clinically, relates to the increased intraglomerular hydrostatic pressure in patients with hypertensive nephrosclerosis (i.e. the Brenner hypothesis). Thus, both afferent and efferent glomerular arteriolar constriction occurs in patients with prolonged systemic arterial hypertension, with renal parenchymal involvement favouring elevated glomerular hydrostatic capillary pressure, glomerular ultrafiltration of protein, and consequent hyalinosis and glomerulosclerosis. With therapeutic reduction of afferent and efferent arteriolar resistance (with angiotensin-converting enzyme inhibitors or angiotensin II receptor blockade), glomerular hydrostatic pressure will also diminish in association with reduced filtered protein and reversal or inhibition of further progression of glomerular sclerosis (see Chapter 6). These findings provide credibility to the concept that angiotensin II participates in the progression of nephrosclerosis in essential hypertension as well as in diabetic renal disease; they also strongly suggest that inhibition of angiotensin II confers significant benefit to these patients.

Fluid volume partitions

As originally postulated by Starling, local haemodynamic and other pressure alterations are responsible for the movement of water across the major body fluid compartments (**1.3**). These factors include the local capillary hydrostatic and local tissue pressures as well as the protein oncotic pressures, intravascularly and extravascularly. In general, total body water is normal in essential hypertension and seems to be normally distributed between the extracellular and intracellular fluid compartments. However, although there is much epidemiological evidence suggesting deranged sodium handling in patients with hypertension, there is little evidence supporting the concept that total body sodium is increased in hypertensive disease or that it is associated with expanded total body water or, even, increased blood pressure sensitivity. In contrast, emerging data suggest other effects of sodium excess on heart, aorta, kidney, and vessels. In addition, there is good clinical investigative evidence that the extracellular fluid volume may be maldistributed in hypertension. Thus, as intravascular (i.e. plasma) volume becomes contracted in patients with essential hypertension, it may be associated with greater interstitial fluid volume. This movement of fluid from the intravascular to the extravascular (including interstitial) fluid compartments has specific pathophysiological implications (**1.7**).

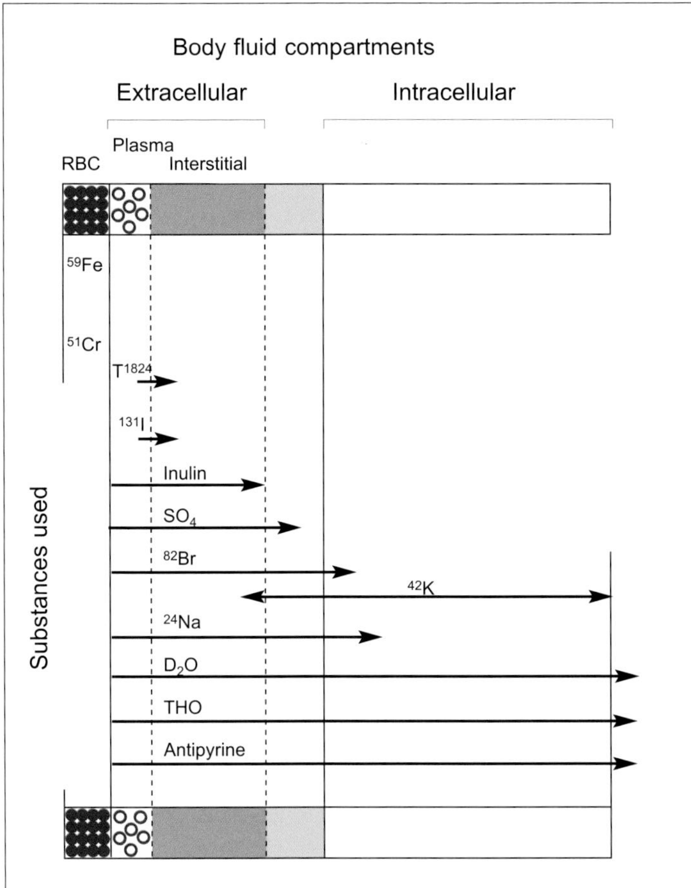

1.7 Extracellular and intracellular body fluid compartments and the various labels used to determine them quantitatively.

Sodium metabolism

As suggested above, many epidemiological studies have demonstrated a direct correlation between the magnitude of dietary sodium intake and the prevalence of hypertension in many populations. Other studies have shown that in those societies with daily sodium dietary intakes of <60 mmol (mEq), hypertension is practically non-existent and these populations fail to show a rise in arterial pressure with ageing. Furthermore, still other epidemiological studies have demonstrated that there may be genetically determined alterations in sodium transport across cell membranes in different populations of patients with essential hypertension.

Notwithstanding the abundance of the above epidemiological data supporting an important role for the sodium ion in essential hypertension, there is a relative paucity of pathophysiological data confirming this thesis clinically. Indeed, only about one-third of patients with hypertension demonstrate increased pressure responsiveness to sodium (i.e. salt) loading. The major problem lies in the elusive ability to define just which patients with essential hypertension are sodium sensitive and those which are not. The best proof in the individual patient is to restrict sodium intake to see if blood pressure becomes reduced. The subject currently remains one of great controversy. As we describe later, salt excess is associated with structural and functional derangements of the target organs of the disease.

Hormonal alterations

Because of the controversial role of sodium in essential hypertension, many studies have focused upon the role of adrenal corticosteroids and their regulatory genes in the pathogenesis of hypertension in at least some patients. There have been very few patients with essential hypertension who have demonstrated an abnormality of steroidal mechanisms underlying the hypertension disease process. In general, aldosterone seems to be synthesized, released, and excreted in proportion to the levels of stimulation of the renin–angiotensin system in patients with essential hypertension; there does not seem to be any clear-cut derangement in adrenal steroid biosynthesis in such patients. In those patients with abnormalities in steroidal biosynthesis and release, the derangements are due to specific adrenal diseases (Cushing's syndrome and disease, primary hyperaldosteronism, hydroxylase and other enzyme deficiencies). Recent studies in many of these secondary hypertensions have demonstrated specific genetic enzymatic abnormalities that account for the steroidal defect. Hormonal alterations have been demonstrated in other patients with hypertension (*Table 1.4*).

Neural mechanisms

The autonomic nervous system normally participates in the control of arterial pressure; this role may be altered in patients with essential hypertension. One would normally expect that, as arterial pressure increases, heart rate should slow. However, most patients with essential hypertension demonstrate a faster resting heart rate than normal. This is but one manifestation of the phenomenon of the 'resetting' or altered baroreceptor sensitivity in hypertension. In addition, increased release, sensitivity, and excretion of norepinephrine (noradrenaline) has been repeatedly demonstrated in patients with essential hypertension and, more frequently, in patients with borderline or earlier stages of the disease. These findings have been supported by the demonstration of increased serum catecholamine concentration in proportion to the altered haemodynamics in these patients. The elevation of serum catecholamine concentration in these patients, however, is not nearly as high as in patients with phaeochromocytoma.

It is of interest that in patients with less severe essential hypertension, particularly those with a hyperdynamic beta-adrenergic circulatory state (with or without idiopathic mitral valve prolapse syndrome), serum norepinephrine (noradrenaline) concentration is frequently elevated. This finding provides one explanation for the altered haemodynamic findings as well as the augmented myocardial contractility, the idiopathic mitral valve prolapse, and the associated cardiac dysrhythmias. In general, there have been no alterations reported in catecholamine biosynthesis or in release or reuptake of these substances, although increased responsiveness of beta-adrenergic receptor sites has been reported (see Chapter 5). Furthermore, the reported altered responses to upright tilting, Valsalva manoeuvres, and tyramine stimulation of norepinephrine (noradrenaline) release from nerve endings may provide a useful indication of adrenergic neural participation in certain patients with essential hypertension.

Several years ago, the clonidine suppression test was introduced to differentiate patients with phaeochromocytoma from those patients with essential hypertension (who demonstrate smaller elevations of plasma catecholamines). Clonidine (a centrally acting adrenergic inhibitor) administration will suppress elevated catecholamine levels to normal levels in patients with essential hypertension but not in those with phaeochromocytoma.

Renopressor system

The enzyme renin is released from the juxtaglomerular apparatus of the kidney through several mechanisms (*Table 1.7*). Renin acts on its circulating peptide substrate angiotensinogen, produced in the liver, resulting in the generation of the pressor octapeptide angiotensin II (**1.8**). The octapeptide apparently generates other peptides whose actions are under active investigation. Angiotensin II has a number of sites of action, most notably in blood vessels and adrenal cortex, to produce vasoconstriction and aldosterone release, respectively. In addition, angiotensin is also generated locally in heart, vessels, kidneys, and other organs with specific local actions (*Table 1.8*). The precise roles for these local systems are not yet clearly known but intracellular generation of angiotensin II affects muscle protein synthesis, with inherent implications relating to the development or reversal of vascular and ventricular hypertrophy. Local generation of angiotensin II may be of particular importance in: (a) the function of the cardiac or arteriolar myocyte which produces the peptide (an intracrine function); (b) the effect on neighbouring cells (an autocrine function); or (c) association with other hormones (e.g. kinins, catecholamines, atrial natriuretic peptide, endothelin) within that organ (a paracrine function) (**1.9**).

Table 1.7 Mechanisms of increased renin release from the kidney

- Reduced renal blood flow and/or perfusion pressure
- Contracted intravascular volume
- Dietary sodium restriction (<100 mmol [mEq]/day)
- Increased beta-adrenergically mediated neural input
- Reduced aldosterone levels in blood
- Upright posture
- Hormones or humoral agents (e.g. catecholamines)
- Drugs (e.g. diuretics)

Table 1.8 Sites of action of angiotensin II

Site	*Action*
Vascular smooth muscle	Vasoconstriction
Adrenal medulla	Release of catecholamines
Adrenal cortex	Aldosterone
Medulla of brain	Thirst
Medullary centres	Augment adrenergic outflow
Paravertebral ganglia	Augment norepinephrine (noradrenaline) release
Local synthesis of angiotensin II in:	
Heart	Myocytic hypertrophy, fibrosis, apoptosis
Brain	Adrenergic outflow
Arteries	Myocytic hypertrophy, fibrosis
Other organs (uterus, liver, salivary glands)	To be resolved

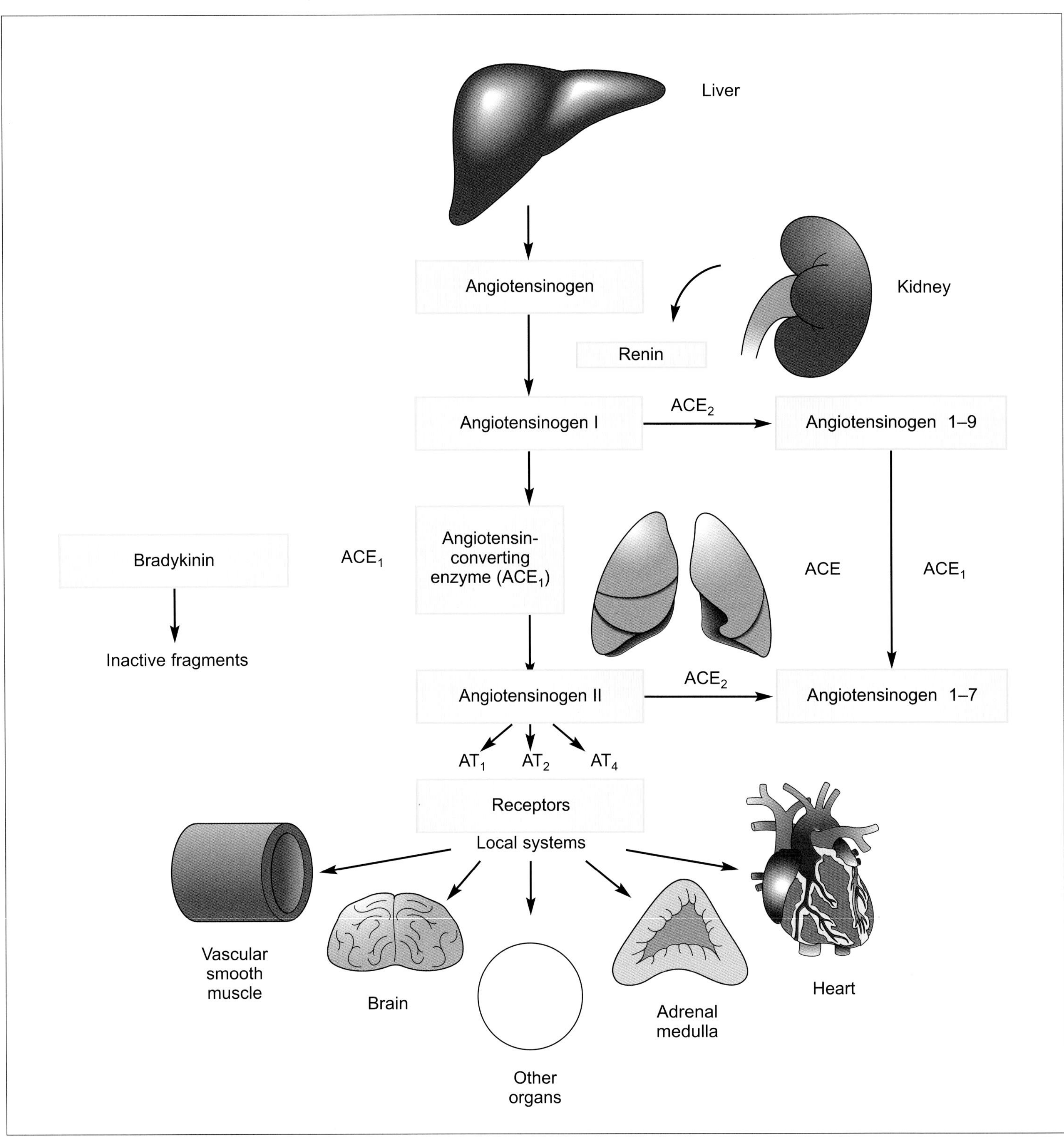

1.8 Generation of angiotensin II: the classical endocrine renin–angiotensin system.

Measurement of plasma renin activity (PRA) has important clinical implications not only in the classification of patients with essential hypertension, but in other hypertensive diseases including renal arterial disease and steroidal forms of hypertension (see Chapters 2, 6 and 7).

Much interest has been engendered in recent years about

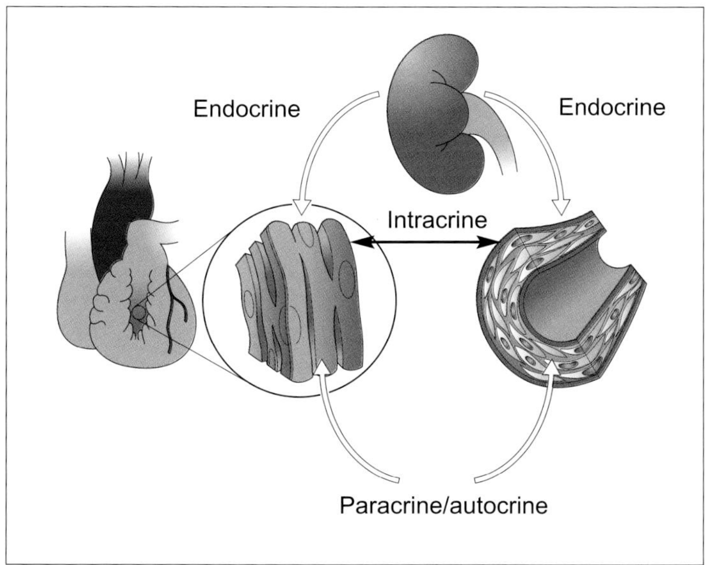

1.9 Systemic and local renin–angiotensin systems.

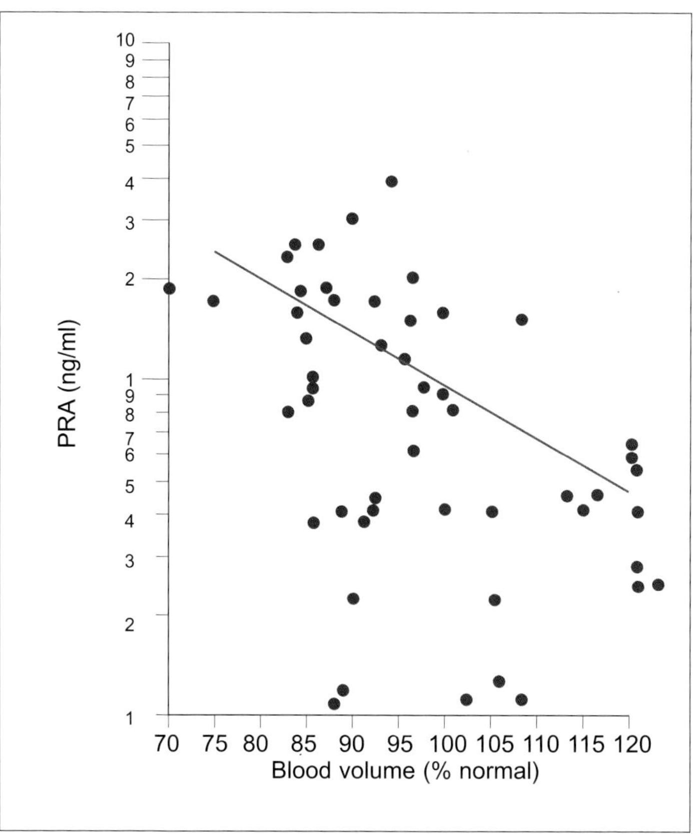

1.10 Plasma renin vs. blood volume in normal men and men with essential hypertension.

the role of the renin–angiotensin system in patients with essential hypertension. Laragh and his colleagues have suggested that patients with essential hypertension may be classified (or 'profiled') according to the levels of PRA, expressed with respect to 24-hour sodium excretion. PRA can be increased in those patients with reduced dietary sodium intake (<100 mmol [mEq]) and, conversely, PRA will be reduced in those patients with excessive dietary sodium intake. This categorization has been used not only conceptually with respect to the pathophysiological alterations, but also for selecting antihypertensive therapy on a physiological basis. Thus, those patients with high PRA may be at increased risk of premature cardiovascular events, stroke, other morbidity, and death. In contrast, those patients with low PRA may be at less risk. No precise physiological mechanism has been offered to explain this association. However, it is known that the higher the arterial pressure and the more severe the vascular disease, the greater will be the total peripheral resistance. Consequently, a more contracted intravascular volume will result, and the more contracted the intravascular volume, the greater will be the PRA (**1.10**). With contraction of intravascular volume, blood and plasma viscosities also increase; this could be expressed on a microcirculatory level in the coronary or cerebral circulation by augmented protein concentration (including fibrinogen levels) and, hence, greater predisposition for thrombosis.

It is particularly pertinent at this point to consider that hormones, vasoactive substances, and other chemicals and growth factors not only act at their own 'classical' target organs, but also may modify the actions of other blood- or neurally borne or local substances. In this fashion, certain agents may exert their physiological actions most subtly by acting in concert with other substances. It is well known, for example, that angiotensin II can augment or amplify adrenergic function by its interaction with norepinephrine (noradrenaline) at certain brain centres, as well as at peripheral ganglionic or postganglionic sites. Angiotensin may also interact with kinins and prostaglandins in kidney, with atrial peptides at nerve endings, on the cardiac myocyte at the vascular smooth muscle membrane, and with other peptides (e.g. endothelin, neuropeptide Y, substance P) at the vascular smooth muscle membrane or intracellularly. Another possible example of this modulatory cardiovascular action occurs with L-arginine, nitric oxide, and bradykinin at the endothelial level to alter local haemodynamic functions. Endothelial dysfunction (i.e. impaired nitric oxide synthesis) occurs in hypertension, cardiac failure, atherosclerosis, obesity, diabetes mellitus, ageing, cigarette smoking, hyperlipidaemia, and in postmenopausal women not receiving oestrogen replacement therapy. These dysfunctions may be modified by agents that are used to manage these conditions and, hence, may reverse endothelial dysfunction.

Further reading

Ross RC, Bowen-Pope DP, Raines EW: Platelets, macrophages, endothelium, and growth factors. Their effects upon cells and their possible roles in atherogenesis. In: *Atherosclerosis.* KT Lee (ed). *Annals N.Y. Acad. Sci.* 1985;**454**:254–260. *The first report demonstrating that the initial functional derangement of the ventricle (myocytic stretch) initiates the process of hypertrophy through stimulating DNA-mediated protein synthesis. It provides a model for many subsequent studies.*

Libby P, Warner SJC, Salomon RN, Birinyi LK: Production of platelet-derived growth factor-like mitogen by smooth muscle cells from human atheroma. *N. Engl. J. Med.* 1988;**318**:1493–1498.

Sarzani R, Arnaldi G, Takasaki 1, Brecher P, Chobanian AV: Effects of hypertension and aging on platelet-derived growth factor and platelet-derived growth factor receptor expression in rat aorta and heart. *Hypertension* 1991;**18**(Suppl. 111):93–99.

These two references provide excellent discussions on how local vascular growth factors participate in atherogenesis. Most interestingly, these mitogenic factors in atherosclerosis may be the same factors that participate in hypertension, thereby offering a conceptual explanation as to how one disease exacerbates the other.

Page IH: *Hypertension Mechanisms.* Grune and Stratton, Orlando, FL; 1987.

Page IH: Pathogenesis of arterial hypertension. *J.A.M.A.* 1949;**140**:451–458.

Frohlich ED: (State of the Art): The first Irvine H. Page lecture: The mosaic of hypertension: past, present, and future. *J. Hypertension* 1988;**6**(Suppl. 4):S2–S11. *These three references provide discussions on the mosaic concept of Page relating to the multifactorial nature of hypertension and left ventricular hypertrophy.*

Frohlich ED, Apstein C, Chobanian AV, *et al.*: The heart in hypertension. *N. Engl. J. Med.* 1992;**327**:998–1008. *Summary of the heart in hypertension by working group of the National Heart, Lung, and Blood Institute.*

Frohlich ED, Kozul Vj, Tarazi RC, Dustan HP: Physiological comparison of labile and essential hypertension. *Circ. Res.* 1970;**27**(1):55–69.

Frohlich ED, Tarazi RC, Dustan HP: Clinical-physiological correlations in the development of hypertensive heart disease. *Circulation* 1971;**44**:446–455.

Dunn FG, Chandraratna P, de Carvalho JGR, Basta LL, Frohlich ED: Pathophysiologic assessment of hypertensive heart disease with echocardiography. *Am. J. Cardiol.* 1977;**39**:789–795. *These three references are clinical pathophysiological studies describing the development of labile and essential hypertension. The third reference provides that first support to the former discussions on the clinical, structural, and functional progression of hypertensive heart disease.*

Tarazi RC, Dustan HP, Frohlich ED, Gifford RW Jr, Hoffman GC: Plasma volume and chronic hypertension. Relationship to arterial pressure levels in different hypertensive diseases. *Arch. Intern. Med.* 1970;**125**:835–842.

Tarazi RC: Haemodynamic role of extracellular fluid volume. *Circ. Res.* 1976; **38**(Suppl 11):73–83.

Dustan HP, Tarazi RC, Frohlich ED: Functional correlates of plasma renin activity in hypertensive patients. *Circulation* 1970;**41**:555–567. *These three references are studies that develop the concept of fluid volume alterations in clinical hypertensionand the functional correlates of PRA in patients with essential hypertension.*

Sealeyj E, Laragh JH: The renin–angiotensin–aldosterone system for normal regulation of blood pressure and sodium and potassium homeostasis. In: *Hypertension: Pathophysiology, Diagnosis, and Management.* JH Laragh, BM Brenner (eds). Raven Press, New York, 1990, pp.1287–1317.

Bühler FR, Laragh JH, Baer L, Vaughan ED Jr, Brunner HR: Propranolol inhibition of renin secretion: a specific approach to diagnosis and treatment of renin-dependent hypertensive diseases. *N. Engl. J. Med.* 1972;**287**:1209–1214. *These references introduce the concept and therapeutic rationale for the profiling of PRA in hypertension.*

Alderman MH, Madhavan S, Ooi WL, Cohan H, Sealey JE, Laragh JH: Association of the renin sodium profile with the risk of myocardial infarction in patients with hypertension. *N. Engl. J. Med.* 1991;**324**:1098–1104. *This reference and Bohler et al. (1972) profile PRA to hypertensive outcomes.*

Chapter 2

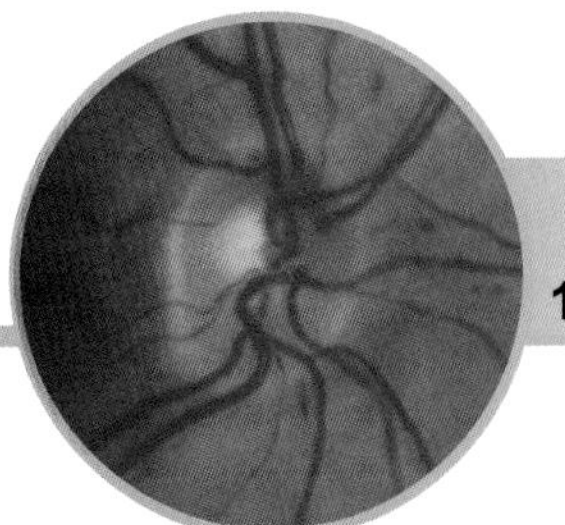

Evaluation of the patient

Introduction

As with all clinical problems, it is essential to evaluate the patient thoroughly before considering management and treatment. If therapy is initiated before overall clinical evaluation has been performed, important clues may be obscured. Consider, for example, the patient with systemic arterial hypertension currently taking as simple a treatment as a thiazide diuretic. Associated metabolic changes may distort the clinical picture, including biochemical and cardiovascular risk factors (*Table 2.1*). This chapter considers important clues that may be obtained from a careful personal and family history, physical examination, and basic laboratory evaluation.

Table 2.1 Biochemical and other risk factors affecting patient evaluation when receiving a thiazide diuretic

Biochemical
- Increased serum concentration of:
  - Creatinine
  - Glucose
  - Cholesterol
  - Uric acid
  - Calcium
- Decrease serum concentration of:
  - Potassium
  - Magnesium

Other risk factors
- Diabetes mellitus
- Hyperlipidaemia
- Hyperuricaemia
- Hypertension, curable causes
- Elevated serum C-reactive protein

Family history

One striking feature of the concept of hypertension as a multifactorial disease is the presence of a strong family history of hypertension in some patients. When there is a family history of hypertension or of premature cardiovascular death, the likelihood of secondary forms of hypertension may be less (*Table 2.2*). However, should any of the secondary forms of hypertension be established, it is possible that the patient may also have essential hypertension, since the latter is present in about 20% of the overall population. Hence, it is important to search for and control other important cardiovascular risk factors, particularly in patients with a family history of premature death (*Table 2.3*). Should hypertension occur in both parents, there are additional considerations; since hypertension is a polygenetic disease, there is a greater likelihood that the disease may be more complex and severe.

Table 2.2 Clues suggesting a diagnosis of secondary hypertension

- Absence of a family history of hypertension
- Sudden onset of hypertension in a child or older adult
- Sudden appearance of an elevated pressure when pressure had been well controlled previously
- Appearance of refractoriness to previous effective antihypertensive therapy
- Physical examination findings or abnormal laboratory findings suggestive of a secondary cause of hypertension

Table 2.3 Important factors in the family history

Family history of premature death from
- Myocardial infarction
- Heart failure
- Stroke
- Kidney failure

Coexistent risk factors with hypertension
- Atherosclerosis
- Obesity
- Diabetes mellitus
- Hypercholesterolaemia or other hyperlipidaemias
- Gout
- Smoking
- Physical inactivity
- Microalbuminuria
- Age (male ≥55 years; female ≥65 years)
- Black race

Clinical history

In most patients with systemic hypertension there are generally no clinical manifestations other than elevated systolic and/or diastolic pressures. Therefore, unless blood pressure is measured in all patients, hypertension will remain unrecognized and untreated, and there will be no further improvement in the control rates of hypertensive disease in any given population.

The most common symptoms traditionally related to hypertension have been fatigue, headache and epistaxis, but these symptoms are among the most common complaints offered by *any* patient seeking medical attention. However, when other symptoms are present, they are more likely to be related to the 'target organ' (i.e. heart, kidneys, brain) of the disease (*Table 2.4*). In this regard, it is important to question the more subtle signs so that the correct diagnosis can be made for those patients with earlier stage 1 hypertension.

Table 2.4 Symptoms of hypertension related to target organ involvement

Brain
- Transitory episode(s) of sensory or motor deficit
- Dizziness, fainting, vertigo
- Sudden loss of vision (total or part of visual field)
- Sudden lancinating vertical headache (ruptured aneurysm)
- Transient sensory motor or speech defects

Cardiovascular
- Diminished exercise tolerance
- Easily fatigued
- Palpitations
- Feeling of 'skipped heartbeats'
- Faster heart rate that persists after exercise ceases
- Chest pain, even in the absence of occlusive coronary disease
- Shortness of breath
- Peripheral oedema
- Heat intolerance or facial or upper chest flushing
- Florid complexion (Gainsböck's syndrome) associated with increased haemoglobin, haematocrit
- Slow to heal skin ulcerations

Kidney
- Nocturia – diminished renal concentrating ability
- Flank pain – suggests renal arterial disease, stones, cystic disease
- Haematuria – arterial disease, glomerulonephritis, cysts, stones
- Appearance of 'foamy' urine
- Sudden flank pain with or without haematuria

Physical examination

Blood pressure measurement

Hypertension cannot be controlled and its complications cannot be prevented if blood pressure is not routinely measured and properly obtained during every physical examination. This should be done by all primary care physicians, specialists, dentists and other health care professionals. However, it is important to emphasize that the diagnosis should not be made on the basis of any single measurement. Repeated measurements should be obtained

Table 2.5 Procedure for the indirect measurement of blood pressure

- Patients should be seated with the arm bared, supported, and at heart level. The patient should not have smoked or ingested caffeine within 30 minutes before measurement
- Measurement should begin after at least 5 minutes of rest. The appropriate cuff size must be used to ensure an accurate measurement. The cuff bladder should nearly (at least 80%) or completely encircle the arm
- Measurements should be taken with a mercury sphygmomanometer, a recently calibrated aneroid manometer or a calibrated electronic device
- Both the systolic and diastolic pressure should be recorded. Disappearance of sound (phase V) should be used for the diastolic reading
- Two or more readings separated by 2 minutes must be taken and an average reading obtained. If the first two readings differ by >5 mmHg, additional readings must be obtained
- In addition, blood pressure must be measured in both arms on the initial physical examination and periodically thereafter. It is not unusual that the measured pressure will be reduced over several years from the initial examination in those elderly patients with occlusive brachial arterial disease
- During the procedure the patient and examiner should refrain from talking

during each individual examination, and the diagnosis is established if these blood pressure measurements are made two or three times, and were elevated on three successive office visits (including the first). The American Heart Association, the Joint National Committee and the World Health Organization have all recommended similar follow-up procedures for repeated measurements based upon the initial measurements.

These recommendations advise use of a systematic technique (*Table 2.5*) and additionally advise on the purpose and meaning of blood pressure measurements, with specific recommendations on follow-up. Furthermore, should the patient assist in follow-up with home blood pressure measurements, the instrument must be calibrated and validated periodically (at least once annually). There is no part of the physical examination on which the diagnosis of hypertension is more dependent than the precise and repeated measurement of blood pressure.

Ophthalmoscopy

The small vessels of the optic fundus provide an excellent means for assessing the degree of systemic vasoconstriction (**2.1A–F**). This examination should be performed routinely. The earliest stage (group 1) of hypertensive vascular disease is recognized by increased tortuosity and mild constriction of the vessels. Coexisting sclerotic changes are manifested by the discontinuity of the vessels at the arteriovenous (AV) crossings (i.e. AV nicking (group 2)(**2.1B**). The appearance of exudates and haemorrhages (group 3) signals accelerated hypertension; and with the appearance of papilloedema (group 4), malignant hypertension is established (**2 .1C–F**).

The American Ophthalmological Association has offered a more detailed classification based upon the degree of narrowing of both the retinal arterioles and venules (*Table 2.6*).

Peripheral pulses

The femoral and brachial arterial pulsations in all patients with hypertension must be compared in order to search for any delay in the propagation of the aortic pulse wave, suggesting the presence of aortic coarctation (particularly in younger patients). Although this diagnosis should be considered in all patients, including adults, it may also suggest an atherosclerotic occlusive process in the elderly, particularly if there are asymmetrical brachial arterial pressures or if, on long-term follow-up, there is an unexplained reduction in pressure taken in one arm, or a reduction or loss of peripheral pulsations. If that occurs, pressure should be measured in the contralateral arm, and further evaluation can be done for occlusive vascular disease.

Auscultation of the carotid arteries for systolic bruits may provide signs of preventable strokes and transient ischaemic attacks (especially if associated with neurological signs and symptoms). It is important to dissociate bruits heard over the carotid arteries from transmission of aortic systolic ejection-type murmurs. This usually can be clarified by listening carefully for the timing and character of the bruits. Furthermore, funduscopy may reveal cholesterol emboli in the retinal arterioles. Renal arterial bruits on examination of the abdomen, flanks and back provide an important sign of renovascular hypertension. Systolic bruits are more commonly detected, especially in older patients, and may not be associated solely with occlusive renal arterial disease.

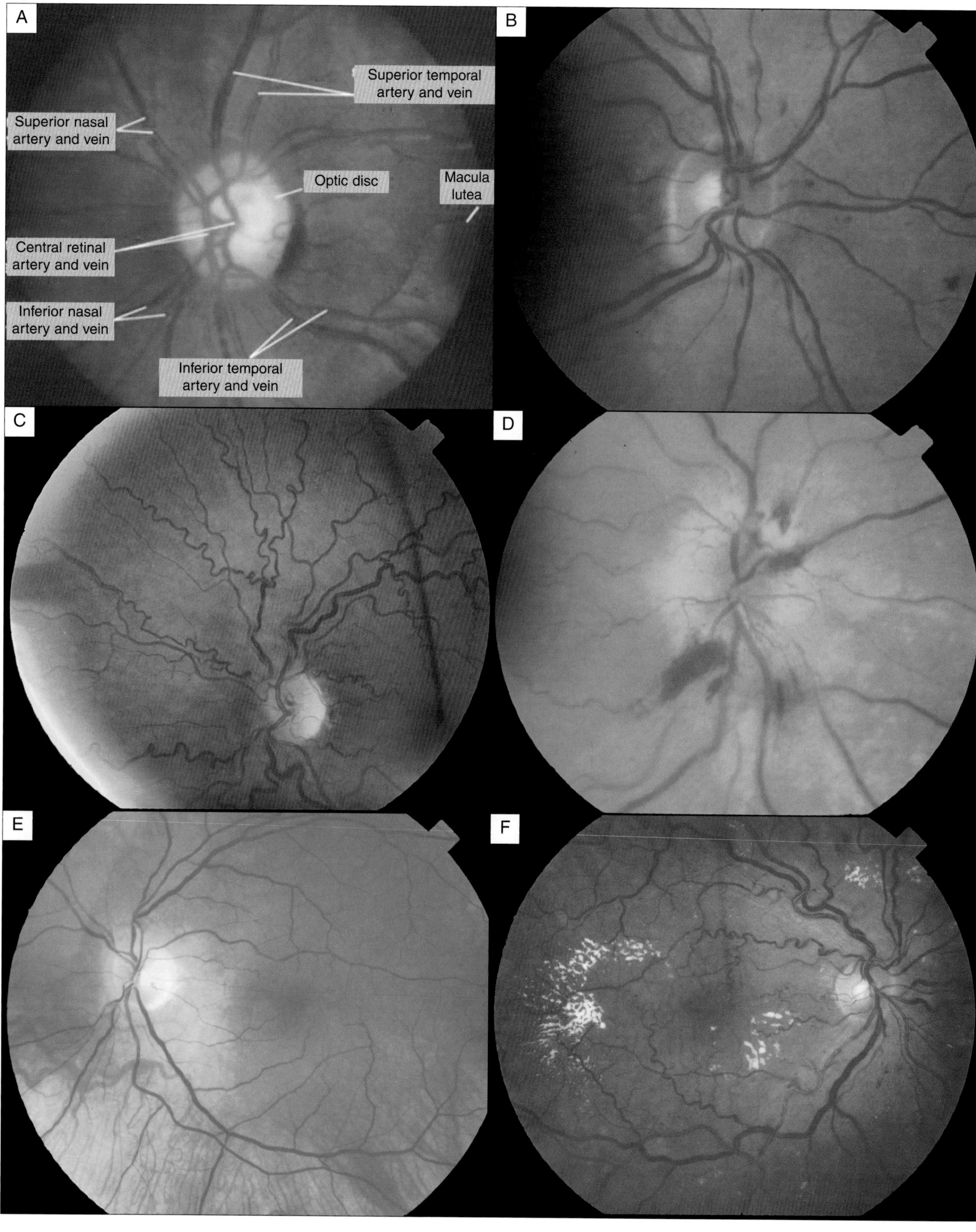
A
B
C
D
E
F
Superior temporal artery and vein
Superior nasal artery and vein
Optic disc
Macula lutea
Central retinal artery and vein
Inferior nasal artery and vein
Inferior temporal artery and vein

2.1 Fundoscopy in hypertension. **A**: normal funduscopic examination demonstrating vessels and the optic nerve head; **B**: severe arteriolar constriction; **C**: marked arteriolar tortuosity; **D**: marked arteriolar constriction and flame-shaped haemorrhages; **E**: accelerated hypertension with severe arteriolar constriction, haemorrhages and exudates; **F**: malignant hypertension with severe arteriolar constriction and tortuosity, haemorrhages, exudates and papilloedema.

Table 2.6 Classification of hypertensive retinopathy

Keith–Wagener–Barker classification
- Group I – tortuosity, minimal constriction
- Group II – as above + arteriovenous nicking
- Group III – as above + haemorrhages and exudates
- Group IV – papilloedema

American Ophthalmological Society Committee Classification (Wagener–Clay–Gipner)
Generalized arteriolar constriction:
- Grade 1 – arterioles $^3/_4$ of normal calibre; AV ratio of 1:2
- Grade 2 – arterioles $^1/_2$ of normal calibre; AV ratio of 1:3
- Grade 3 – arterioles $^1/_3$ of normal calibre; AV ratio of 1:4
- Grade 4 – arterioles thread-like or invisible

Focal arteriolar constriction or sclerosis
- Grade 1 – localized arteriolar narrowing to $^2/_3$ calibre of proximal segment
- Grade 2 – localized arteriolar narrowing to $^1/_2$ calibre of proximal segment
- Grade 3 – localized arteriolar narrowing to $^1/_3$ calibre of proximal segment
- Grade 4 – arterioles invisible beyond focal constriction, arteriolar–venular.

Generalized sclerosis
- Grade 1 – increased light-striping; mild AV nicking
- Grade 2 – coppery arteriolar colour; moderate AV nicking; veins almost completely invisible below arteriolar crossing
- Grade 3 – silver arteriolar colour; severe AV nicking
- Grade 4 – arterioles visible only as fibrous cords without bloodstreams

Haemorrhage and exudates
Grades 1 to 4 (based on the number of affected quadrants divided by 2)

Papilloedema
Grades 1 to 4 (based on dioptres of elevation)

However, when the abdominal bruit is associated with a diastolic component in the upper quadrants of the abdomen or flanks, the possibility of renal arterial disease becomes much more likely and should be focused on.

Cardiac examination

Even before cardiac structure is altered (particularly in young patients), precordial palpation may reveal evidence of functional hyperdynamic cardiac changes, namely hyperdynamic apical impulse and a faster heart rate. As the heart adapts structurally to the increasing afterload by development of left ventricular hypertrophy (LVH), increased ventricular mass may be suspected by a sustained apical lift although it may not be detectable by the chest roentgenogram. The electrocardiogram and echocardiographic assessment are more sensitive. Nevertheless, the earliest clinical index of cardiac involvement in hypertension is left atrial enlargement, which may be suspected by an atrial diastolic gallop (fourth heart sound or the *bruit de gallop*). This finding is highly concordant with at least two of four electrocardiographic criteria of left atrial abnormality (*Table 2.7*, **2.2**).

Table 2.7 Abnormal diagnostic electrocardiographic criteria

Left atrial abnormality – two of four of the following criteria

- P wave in lead II ≥ 0.3 mV and ≥0.12 s
- Bipeak interval in notched P wave ≥ 0.04 s
- Ratio of P wave duration to PR segment ≥1.6 (lead II)
- Terminal atrial forces (in V1) ≥0.04 s

Left ventricular hypertrophy

- Ungerleider index +15% on chest X-ray alone
- Ungerleider index +10% on chest X-ray + two of the following ECG criteria:
  - – Sum of tallest R and deepest S waves ≥4.5 mV (precordial)
  - – LV 'strain' – i.e. QRS and T wave vectors 180° apart
  - – QRS frontal axis <0°
  - – All three of ECG criteria above

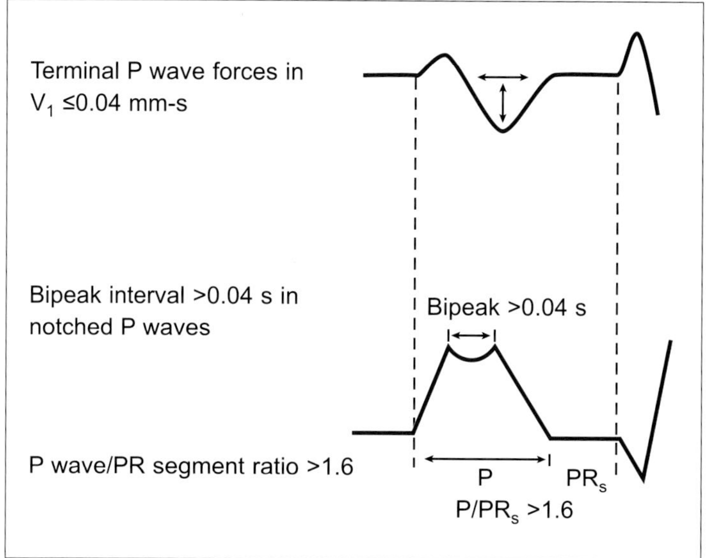

2.2 Electrocardiographic criteria for left atrial abnormality.

Haemodynamic and echocardiographic studies have demonstrated that when electrocardiographic evidence of left atrial abnormality is present (even without other indications of LVH), there is adequate evidence of impaired left ventricular (LV) systolic function. As LVH becomes more evident clinically, as indicated above, there is palpable evidence of a sustained LV lift (or 'heave') and further impairment of contractile function. In patients with severe LVH, the presence of a third heart sound (ventricular diastolic gallop) eventually connotes the presence of early LV failure. In those patients with a very high arterial pressure, an aortic diastolic 'blowing' murmur may occur as the result of a functional eversion of the aortic cusp by elevated pressure and total peripheral resistance. The more frequently heard precordial or vascular systolic ejection murmur suggests either outflow tract obstruction from (absolute or relative) aortic stenosis (associated with ageing), or a haemic murmur related to a hyperkinetic circulation or coexistent anaemia.

Other physical findings

The so-called 'buffalo hump,' seen on the back below the neck, suggests Cushing's syndrome (**2.3**). This may also be associated with abdominal striae and girdle obesity. Neurofibromatosis or café-au-lait skin spots can suggest possible coexistent phaeochromocytoma (**2.4A–C**). In the days prior to effective antihypertensive therapy, cutaneous ulcerations were seen as manifestations of severely impaired cutaneous blood flow (**2.5**). Appearance of anaemia on physical examination in the black patient should suggest coexistent haemoglobinopathy or anaemia secondary to chronic renal disease. Careful abdominal examination is necessary for the auscultation of bruits, as well as for the presence of the palpable kidneys of polycystic kidney disease (PKD). When the latter occurs, hepatic cysts, secondary polycythaemia and cerebral aneurysmal disease of the circle of Willis should also be considered.

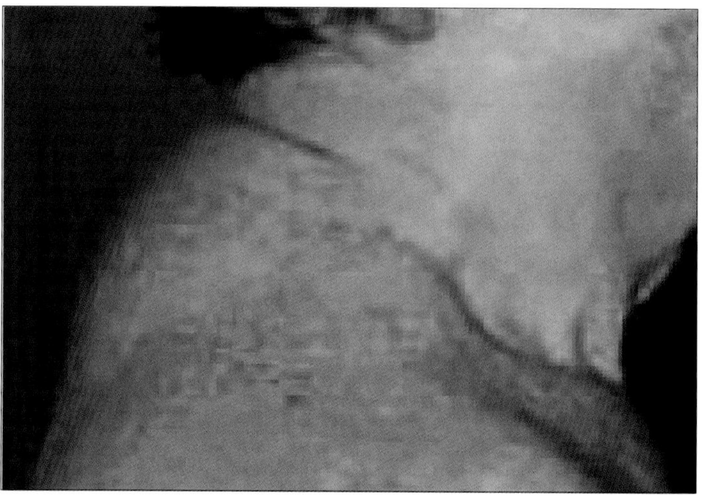

2.3 Buffalo hump.

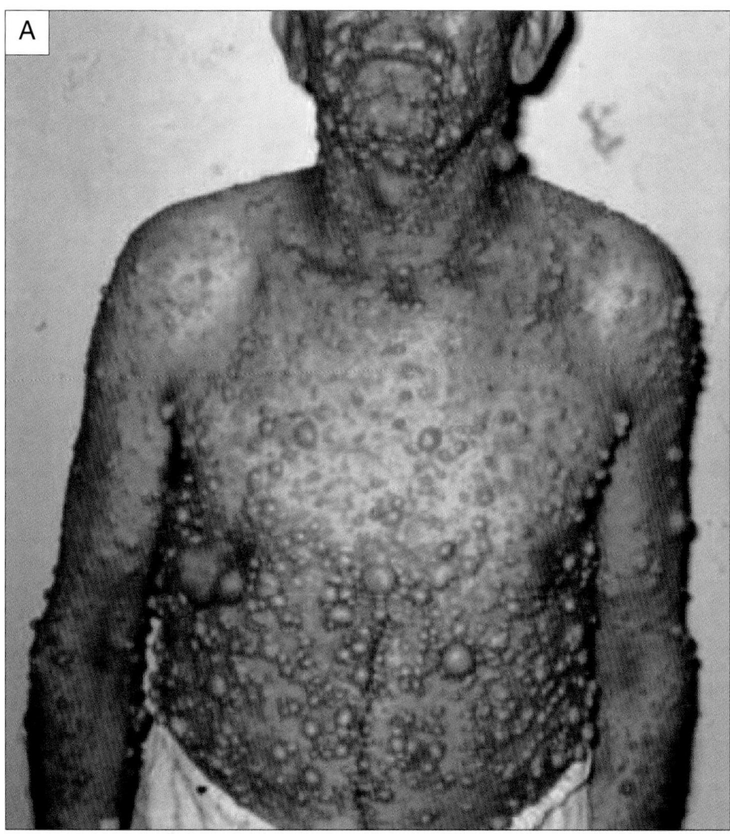

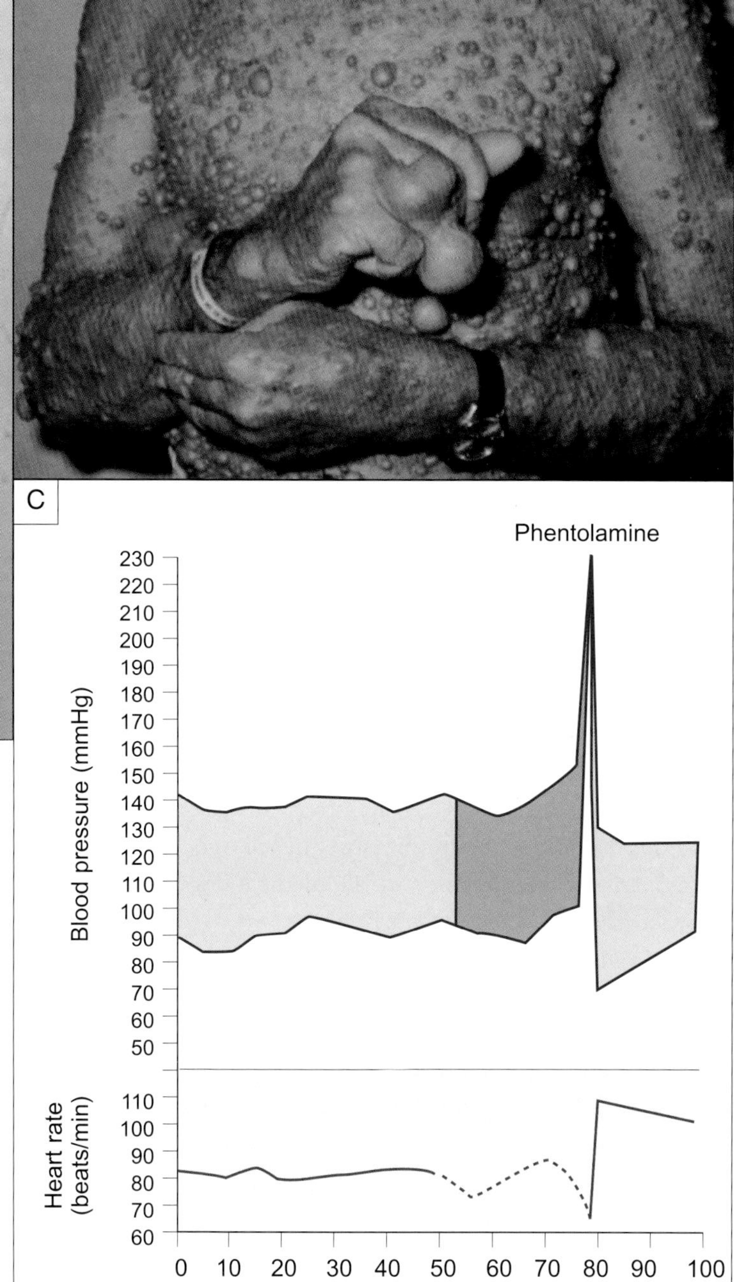

2.4 Neurofibromatosis. **A**, **B:** skin lesions; **C**: patients may also have a phaeochromocytoma. When the angiotensin II anatagonist saralasin is infused it stimulates the release of catecholamines from the phaeochromocytoma. Medullary blood pressure is reduced with administration of the adrenergic antagonist phentolamine. The phaeochromocytoma was subsequently surgically removed.

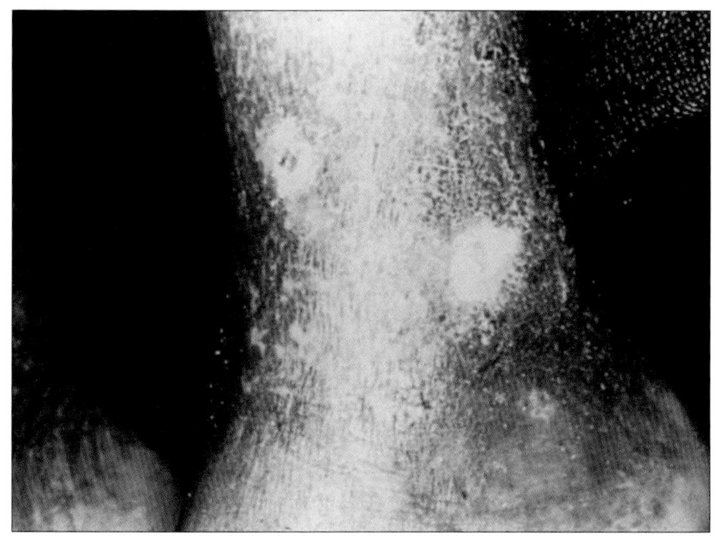

2.5 Hypertension-related cutaneous skin ulceration. The lesion was slow healing but improved with blood pressure control.

Laboratory studies

It is important to discuss with the patient appropriate preparation for laboratory tests, including cessation of all medication, preferably for at least 2 weeks (*Table 2.8*). Even a sodium-restricted diet may stimulate adrenal cortical production of aldosterone in sufficient quantities to suggest a state of hyperaldosteronism. Dietary sodium intake in excess of 100 mmol (mEq)/day (2.3 g), will obviate this possibility. This degree of restriction of daily sodium intake may still be effective, either in reducing pressure in some patients or in enhancing effectiveness of the antihypertensive drugs.

It is important to realize that diuretics, laxatives and intercurrent gastrointestinal problems (associated with nausea, vomiting and diarrhoea) may incur sufficient volume depletion and electrolyte loss so as to produce evidence of secondary hyperaldosteronism with associated hypokalaemia and alkalosis. Some antihypertensive drugs may have effects lasting for several weeks, thereby providing a false concept of 'baseline' untreated pressure levels. For example, the thiazide diuretics may have persistent effects for 2 weeks following discontinuation. Oral contraceptives may elevate arterial pressure and alter intravascular volume, haemodynamics and plasma renin activity. Certain 'street drugs' (e.g. heroin, cocaine) will elevate blood pressure; hence, it is important to obtain an accurate history of all medications or over-the-counter drugs that the patient is taking.

Certainly, not all studies discussed below may be necessary in evaluating all patients; however, this discussion provides a means for understanding overall laboratory evaluation. The minimal evaluation is presented in *Table 2.9*. The fewer the laboratory studies, the more cost-effective the evaluation will be. However, modern automated laboratory testing techniques provide more measurements and thus a more comprehensive evaluation, frequently at no greater cost.

Table 2.8 Laboratory tests for the evaluation hypertension

Blood studies
- Complete blood count
- White blood cell count (and differential)
- Haemoglobin concentration
- Haematocrit
- Adequacy of platelets

Blood chemistries
- Glucose (fasting, 2-hour postprandial, or glucose tolerance test, as indicated)
- Uric acid concentration
- Cholesterol (total and with high- and low-density lipoprotein fractions) and triglyceride concentrations
- Renal function (serum creatinine and/or blood urea concentrations)
- Serum electrolyte (Na, K, Cl, CO_2) concentrations
- Calcium and phosphate concentrations
- Total protein and albumin concentrations
- Hepatic function (alkaline phosphatase, bilirubin, serum glutamic oxaloacetic transaminase, serum glutamic pyruvic transaminase, lactic acid dehydrogenase)
- Glycosylated haemoglobin (HbA1c)
- Thyroid-stimulating hormone
- Prostate-specific antigen (PSA)

Urine
- Urinalysis
- Microalbuminuria
- Urine culture (if history of repeated urinary tract infections)
- 24-hour collection (protein, Na, K, creatinine)

Cardiac examinations
- Electrocardiogram – standard 12-lead
- Limited echocardiogram

Complete blood count (CBC)

In addition to assessing the haematological status of the patient, the CBC has broader significance and importance. If anaemia is present, the physician should determine whether it is a complication of the disease, a side-effect of drug therapy or a result of a coexistent disease (*Table 2.10*). An elevated haemoglobin concentration or haematocrit frequently occurs in patients with essential hypertension (see Gaisböck syndrome, Chapter 1). It is also of value to know pretreatment white blood cell count, since leucopenia may complicate angiotensin-converting enzyme (ACE) therapy. Thus, a baseline haemogram determination may be of great value for future care.

Blood chemistry

Several laboratory tests may be of particular value in evaluating the patient with hypertension (*Table 2.8*). The

Table 2.9 Minimum laboratory evaluation of a patient with hypertension

Blood studies
- Complete blood count
- Serum creatinine and/or blood urea nitrogen concentration
- Serum potassium concentration
- Fasting blood sugar
- Uric acid concentration
- Lipid profile (with low-density and high-density lipoprotein, cholesterol and triglyceride concentrations)
- Serum calcium concentration

Cardiac
- Electrocardiogram (standard 12-lead)

fasting blood glucose concentration may be abnormal since diabetes mellitus and the metabolic syndrome (syndrome X) commonly coexist with hypertension (*Table 2.11*). Alternatively, the fasting blood glucose concentration may be normal but a 2-hour postprandial blood glucose measurement may be elevated, alerting the clinician to other diabetic manifestations.

Furthermore, abnormal carbohydrate tolerance exists in excess of 65% of patients with essential hypertension (a finding known for over 80 years), not infrequently coexisting with hyperinsulinaemia. Each of these factors confers independent risk for increased cardiovascular morbidity and mortality. Insulin hypersensitivity may be related to impaired end-organ responsiveness to insulin, which, in turn, may be related to augmented sympathetic responsiveness. Determination of haemoglobin (Hb) A1c concentration

Table 2.10 Differential diagnosis for anaemia presenting with hypertension

- Renal parenchymal disease with failure
- Coexistent unrelated anaemia
- Haemoglobinopathy or thalassaemia
- Iron deficiency
- Side-effect from treatment (e.g. methyldopa-induced haemolysis or chemotherapy)

Table 2.11 Components of the metabolic syndrome (or syndrome X)

- Hypertension
- Obesity
- Carbohydrate intolerance
- Hyperlipidaemia
- Insulin insensitivity

is extremely valuable in assessing current potential risk of developing diabetic vascular complications: the lower the HbA1c value, the lesser the risk.

The serum uric acid determination should suggest which patients may develop more severe hyperuricaemia, or even clinical gout with diuretic therapy. In addition, hyperuricaemia is extremely common in untreated patients with essential hypertension, and is an independent cardiovascular risk factor. Furthermore, studies from the author's laboratory have shown that the higher the serum uric acid concentration is in uncomplicated essential hypertensive patients, the lower the renal blood flow (**2.6A**)

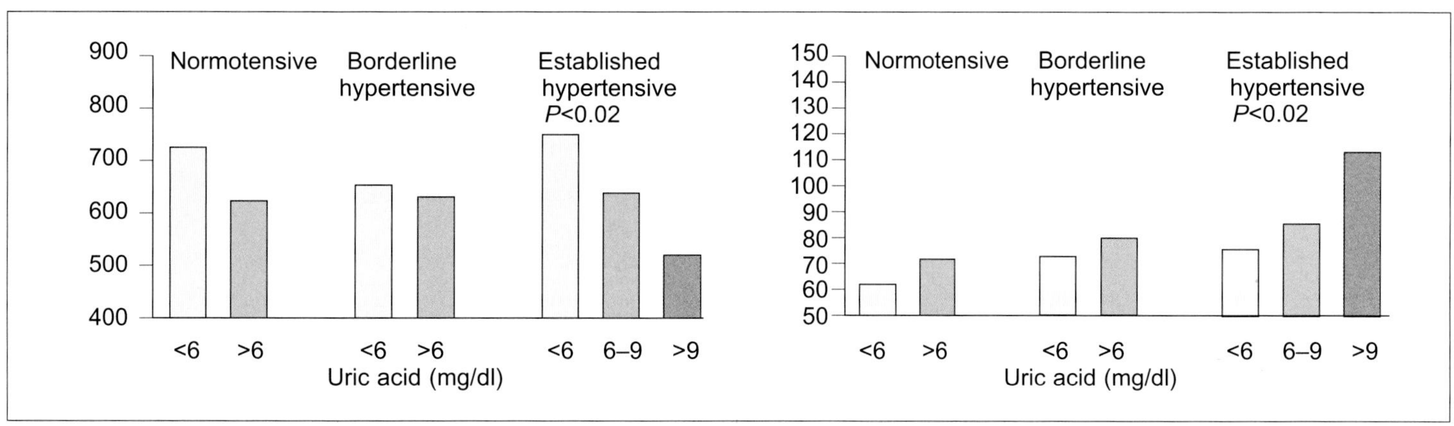

2.6 Relationship between serum uric acid concentration and renal haemodynamics. **A**: the inverse relationship between uric acid concentration and renal blood flow; **B**: the direct relationship between uric acid concentration and renal vascular resistance.

and the higher the renal vascular resistance (**2.6B**). This, then, can be seen in renal haemodynamic functional involvement (i.e. nephrosclerosis) with hypertension. The studies have also shown that the hyperuricaemia and renal haemodynamic alterations follow the earliest echocardiographic changes of LVH, suggesting that early cardiac involvement in hypertension precedes evidence of renal haemodynamic involvement in essential hypertension. When hyperuricaemia occurs (in the untreated patient), intrarenal vascular involvement (i.e. nephrosclerosis) is more likely.

It is essential to assess patients with hypertension for hyperlipidaemia. The serum total cholesterol determination (with high- and low-density lipoprotein cholesterol concentrations), together with measurement of triglyceride concentration, is of major value for controlling yet another risk factor underlying premature coronary heart disease.

The kidney is a prime target organ of hypertension, and renal functional impairment is a major complication. Therefore, it is necessary to determine the serum creatinine concentration (preferably) and/or blood urea nitrogen concentrations in all patients. The author usually obtains both tests. By using the serum creatinine concentration and urinary creatinine excretion (usually 24-hour urinary volume), the creatinine clearance (glomerular filtration rate) can be calculated. Since the prevalence of end-stage renal disease continues to increase, it is vitally important to detect it as early as possible those patients with this potential, since specific antihypertensive therapy and more rigorous control of pressure (<130 mmHg systolic and <80 mmHg diastolic) may delay, if not prevent, its development (see Chapters 2 and 6). Those patients who are at particular risk are black, or have hypertension (with proteinuria or microalbuminuria) or diabetes mellitus.

Measurement of serum electrolyte concentrations, particularly serum potassium, is of great value in excluding diagnostic possibilities of certain secondary forms of hypertension (including those from steroidal hormonal excess and primary or secondary hyperaldosteronism), and the adverse effects of diuretic therapy. In these diseases, the hypokalaemia is associated with alkalosis. Many factors may produce hypokalaemia (*Table 2.12*); conversely, very few factors (other than laboratory error or red cell haemolysis) are responsible for hyperkalaemia. Determination of serum calcium concentration excludes hypercalcaemia, an alteration frequently associated with an increased incidence of hypertension (see Chapter 1). Correction of hypercalcaemia may normalize the abnormally elevated pressure, especially in patients with hyperparathyroidism. Serum magnesium concentration is not a routine test; however, in patients with LVH or cardiac failure with hypokalaemia and cardiac dysrhythmias, it is important to remember that hypomagnesaemia is frequently associated with hypokalaemia.

Routine measurement of serum proteins and hepatic function is usually part of the automated serum chemistry

Table 2.12 Factors involved in hypokalaemia

Dietary sodium excess associated with diuretic therapy

Chronic gastrointestinal potassium losses:
- Vomiting
- Diarrhoea
- Laxative abuse
- Pyloric obstruction
- Nasogastric suction
- Villous adenoma
- Malabsorption syndrome
- Ureterosigmoidostomy

Adrenocortical excess
- Primary aldosteronism (adenoma or hyperplasia)
- Cushing's syndrome or disease
- Other adrenal steroidal hormone excess

Secondary hyperaldosteronism
- Renal arterial disease
- Cirrhosis
- Congestive heart failure

Renal disease (chronic)
- Potassium-wasting nephropathy
- Nephrotic syndrome
- Renal tubular acidosis

Diabetes mellitus (acidosis)

Primary periodic paralysis (hypokalaemic type)

Drug therapy and food
- Diuretics
- Liquorice
- Adrenal steroids
- Salicylate intoxication
- Outdated tetracycline

determinations. Although they may be of little specific value for the patient with hypertension, they may confirm haemoconcentration (i.e. plasma protein concentration) and provide a baseline for later possible coexisting problems (e.g. myocardial infarction, hepatic diseases and statin therapy). Any pharmacological agent might be linked to producing hepatic dysfunction and, when detected, it is important to know whether it is related to drug therapy or a coexistent problem. Measurement of thyroid-stimulating hormone (TSH) is a useful test to evaluate and screen for the possibility of thyroid disease. Finally, while testing for the prostatic screening antigen is not necessary for hypertension, for the overall care of the elderly hypertensive man, this test should be done routinely.

Urinary studies

Of prime importance is routine urinalysis for detection of several comorbid and complicating diseases (*Table 2.13*). Less frequently necessary is a 24-hour urine collection for determining creatinine clearance, assessing dietary sodium intake and potassium wastage (*Table 2.14*). Furthermore, the normal kidney should not excrete >200–300 mg protein daily. Any amount in excess should suggest parenchymal renal disease (including nephrosclerosis) or an effect of the elevated pressure itself (*Table 2.15*).

Nephrosclerosis, *per se*, should not provoke protein excretion >400–500 mg daily. However, if severely elevated arterial pressure is associated with massive proteinuria, proteinuria should decrease with reduction of arterial

Table 2.13 Valuable information obtained from routine urinalysis

Low specific gravity	Impaired urine concentration of advancing nephrosclerosis, parenchymal disease and primary hyperaldosteronism
Alkaline urine	Hyperaldosteronism
Glycosuria	Diabetes mellitus
Abnormal sediment	Renal parenchymal and urinary tract diseases

Table 2.14 Information obtained from 24-hour urine collection

Creatinine	Glomerular filtration rate
Sodium	24-hour sodium intake
Potassium	Primary hyperaldosteronism: • If urinary potassisum excretion is <35 mmol (mEq)/24 h, hypokalaemia of <3.5 mmol (mEq)/l is less likely to be due to primary aldosteronism • If urinary potassium excretion is >50 mmol (mEq)/24 h and K^+ is <3.5 mmol (mEq)/l, then evaluate for primary hyperaldosteronism or another excess adrenal steroid

Table 2.15 Assessment of 24-hour urinary protein excretion

<200 mg/day: normal

>400–500 mg/day: consider nephrosclerosis (if persistent)

>500 mg/day: other causes of renal parenchymal disease (e.g. chronic pyelonephritis; glomerulonephritis) than nephrosclerosis

>2.0–3.0 g/day: consider the causes of nephrotic syndrome

pressure. Microalbuminuria is an important means for assessing early proteinuria, particularly in diabetic patients. With current methodology, the normal range for a normal microalbumin excretion is 30–300 μg per day. Urine culture (and sensitivity) is always wise if there is a likelihood of a urinary tract infection.

Chest X-ray

Although there has been much discussion in recent years on the cost-effectiveness of the routine chest X-ray, it is the author's opinion that this examination is still of great value in the initial evaluation of any patient, especially one with hypertension. This is especially important for the tobacco smoker. It may also be of value in recognizing the presence of LVH (**2.7**), or left ventricular failure (**2.8**). However, once recognized by X-ray, it is likely that such conditions will be demonstrated electrocardiographically and echocardiographically. The Ungerleider index is a very useful means for quantifying the degree of cardiac enlargement (**2.9**). (This technique will provide still more valid information if the films are exposed coincidently with the R wave of the electrocardiogram.) The Ungerleider index takes into consideration the transverse cardiac diameter with respect to the patient's body habitus or height and weight. When the Ungerleider index is ≥15% then that patient is likely to have LVH. This finding has been derived from studies that were correlated with autopsy confirmation. When the Ungerleider index is ≥10% electrocardiographic indices of LVH are found. In addition to detecting an enlarged heart, the chest X-ray is also of value for assessing aortic coarctation (i.e. by costal notching) (**2.10**). Furthermore, the chest film is useful as a baseline study for future evaluation of pulmonary pathology and later complications from hypertension. When obtained, the chest roentgenogram is also useful for detecting substernal thyroid, thymoma, bronchiogenic carcinoma, metastases and other intrapulmonary or skeletal lesions.

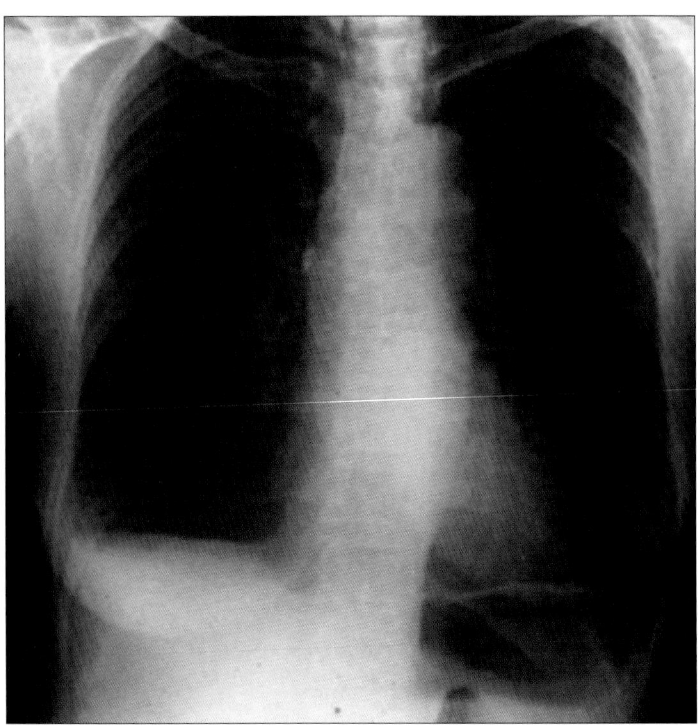

2.7 Chest X-ray of borderline left ventricular enlargement in a hypertensive patient with left ventricular hypertrophy as diagnosed by electrocardiography.

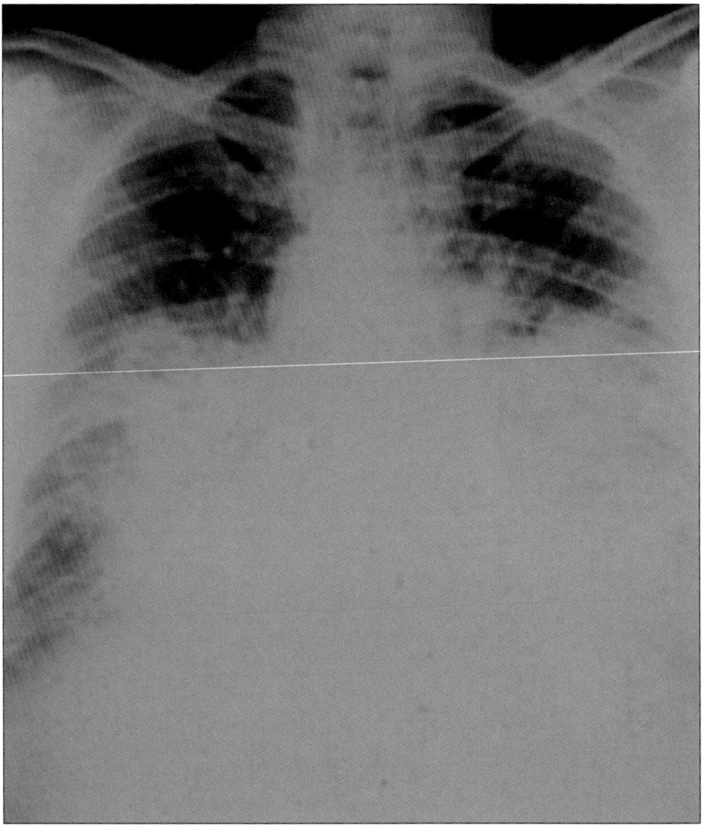

2.8 Chest X-ray in a hypertensive patient with left ventricular hypertrophy and ventricular failure.

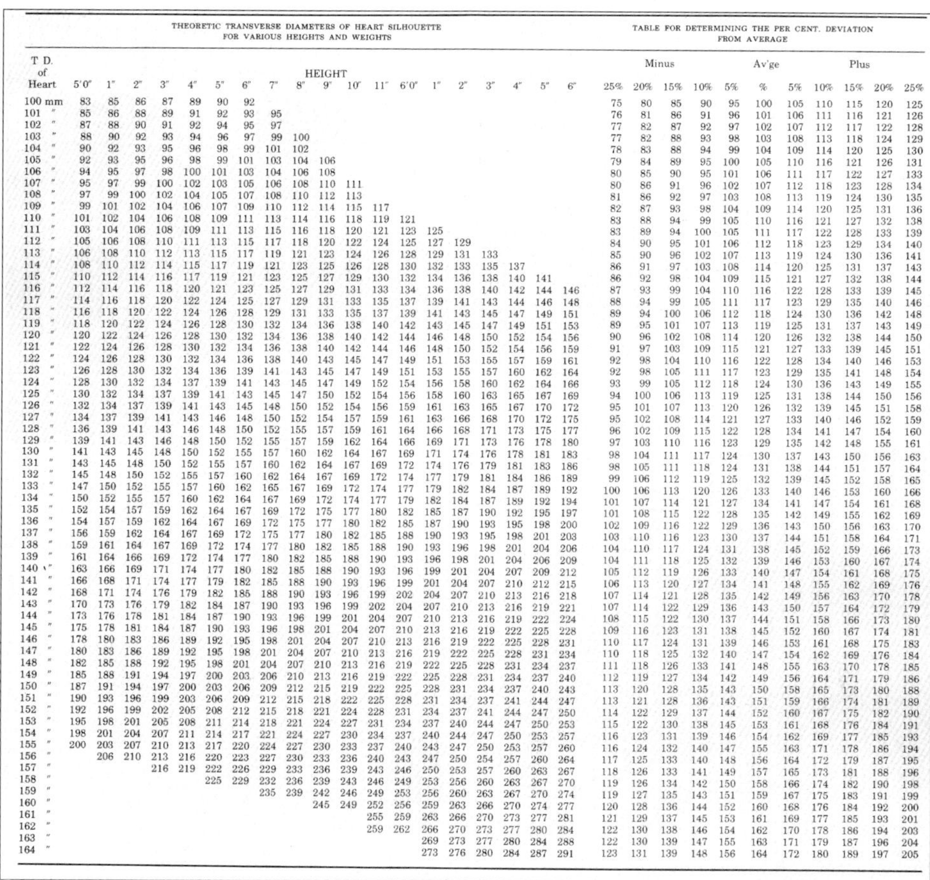

THEORETIC TRANSVERSE DIAMETERS OF HEART SILHOUETTE FOR VARIOUS HEIGHTS AND WEIGHTS

T D. of Heart	HEIGHT 5'0"	1"	2"	3"	4"	5"	6"	7"	8"	9"	10"	11"	6'0"	1"	2"	3"	4"	5"	6"
100 mm	83	85	86	87	89	90	92												
101 "	85	86	88	89	91	92	93	95											
102 "	87	88	90	91	92	94	95	97											
103 "	88	90	92	93	94	96	97	99	100										
104 "	90	92	93	95	96	98	99	101	102										
105 "	92	93	95	96	98	99	101	103	104	106									
106 "	94	95	97	98	100	101	103	104	106	108									
107 "	95	97	99	100	102	103	105	106	108	110	111								
108 "	97	99	100	102	104	105	107	108	110	112	113								
109 "	99	101	102	104	106	107	109	110	112	114	115	117							
110 "	101	102	104	106	108	109	111	113	114	116	118	119	121						
111 "	103	104	106	108	109	111	113	115	116	118	120	121	123	125					
112 "	105	106	108	110	111	113	115	117	118	120	122	124	125	127	129				
113 "	106	108	110	112	113	115	117	119	121	123	124	126	128	129	131	133			
114 "	108	110	112	114	115	117	119	121	123	125	126	128	130	132	133	135	137		
115 "	110	112	114	116	117	119	121	123	125	127	129	130	132	134	136	138	140	141	
116 "	112	114	116	118	120	121	123	125	127	129	131	133	134	136	138	140	142	144	146
117 "	114	116	118	120	122	124	125	127	129	131	133	135	137	139	141	143	144	146	148
118 "	116	118	120	122	124	126	128	129	131	133	135	137	139	141	143	145	147	149	151
119 "	118	120	122	124	126	128	130	132	134	136	138	140	142	143	145	147	149	151	153
120 "	120	122	124	126	128	130	132	134	136	138	140	142	144	146	148	150	152	154	156
121 "	122	124	126	128	130	132	134	136	138	140	142	144	146	148	150	152	154	156	159
122 "	124	126	128	130	132	134	136	138	140	143	145	147	149	151	153	155	157	159	161
123 "	126	128	130	132	134	136	139	141	143	145	147	149	151	153	155	157	160	162	164
124 "	128	130	132	134	137	139	141	143	145	147	149	152	154	156	158	160	162	164	166
125 "	130	132	134	137	139	141	143	145	147	150	152	154	156	158	160	163	165	167	169
126 "	132	134	137	139	141	143	145	148	150	152	154	156	159	161	163	165	167	170	172
127 "	134	137	139	141	143	146	148	150	152	154	157	159	161	163	166	168	170	172	175
128 "	136	139	141	143	146	148	150	152	155	157	159	161	164	166	168	171	173	175	177
129 "	139	141	143	146	148	150	152	155	157	159	162	164	166	169	171	173	176	178	180
130 "	141	143	145	148	150	152	155	157	160	162	164	167	169	171	174	176	178	181	183
131 "	143	145	148	150	152	155	157	160	162	164	167	169	172	174	176	179	181	183	186
132 "	145	148	150	152	155	157	160	162	164	167	169	172	174	177	179	181	184	186	189
133 "	147	150	152	155	157	160	162	165	167	169	172	174	177	179	182	184	187	189	192
134 "	150	152	155	157	160	162	164	167	169	172	174	177	179	182	184	187	189	192	194
135 "	152	154	157	159	162	164	167	169	172	175	177	180	182	185	187	190	192	195	197
136 "	154	157	159	162	164	167	169	172	175	177	180	182	185	187	190	193	195	198	200
137 "	156	159	162	164	167	169	172	175	177	180	182	185	188	190	193	195	198	201	203
138 "	159	161	164	167	169	172	174	177	180	182	185	188	190	193	196	198	201	204	206
139 "	161	164	166	169	172	174	177	180	182	185	188	190	193	196	198	201	204	206	209
140 "	163	166	169	171	174	177	180	182	185	188	190	193	196	199	201	204	207	209	212
141 "	166	168	171	174	177	179	182	185	188	190	193	196	199	201	204	207	210	212	215
142 "	168	171	174	176	179	182	185	188	190	193	196	199	202	204	207	210	213	216	218
143 "	170	173	176	179	182	184	187	190	193	196	199	202	204	207	210	213	216	219	221
144 "	173	176	178	181	184	187	190	193	196	199	201	204	207	210	213	216	219	222	224
145 "	175	178	181	184	187	190	193	196	198	201	204	207	210	213	216	219	222	225	228
146 "	178	180	183	186	189	192	195	198	201	204	207	210	213	216	219	222	225	228	231
147 "	180	183	186	189	192	195	198	201	204	207	210	213	216	219	222	225	228	231	234
148 "	182	185	188	192	195	198	201	204	207	210	213	216	219	222	225	228	231	234	237
149 "	185	188	191	194	197	200	203	206	210	213	216	219	222	225	228	231	234	237	240
150 "	187	191	194	197	200	203	206	209	212	215	219	222	225	228	231	234	237	240	243
151 "	190	193	196	199	203	206	209	212	215	218	222	225	228	231	234	237	241	244	247
152 "	192	196	199	202	205	208	212	215	218	221	224	228	231	234	237	241	244	247	250
153 "	195	198	201	205	208	211	214	218	221	224	227	231	234	237	240	244	247	250	253
154 "	198	201	204	207	211	214	217	221	224	227	230	234	237	240	244	247	250	253	257
155 "	200	203	207	210	213	217	220	224	227	230	233	237	240	243	247	250	253	257	260
156 "		206	210	213	216	220	223	227	230	233	236	240	243	247	250	254	257	260	264
157 "				216	219	222	226	229	233	236	239	243	246	250	253	257	260	263	267
158 "						225	229	232	236	239	243	246	249	253	256	260	263	267	270
159 "								235	239	242	246	249	253	256	260	263	267	270	274
160 "										245	249	252	256	259	263	266	270	274	277
161 "												255	259	263	266	270	273	277	281
162 "												259	262	266	270	273	277	280	284
163 "														269	273	277	280	284	288
164 "														273	276	280	284	287	291

TABLE FOR DETERMINING THE PER CENT. DEVIATION FROM AVERAGE

T D. of Heart	Minus 25%	20%	15%	10%	5%	Av'ge %	Plus 5%	10%	15%	20%	25%
100 mm	75	80	85	90	95	100	105	110	115	120	125
101 "	76	81	86	91	96	101	106	111	116	121	126
102 "	77	82	87	92	97	102	107	112	117	122	128
103 "	77	82	88	93	98	103	108	113	118	124	129
104 "	78	83	88	94	99	104	109	114	120	125	130
105 "	79	84	89	95	100	105	110	116	121	126	131
106 "	80	85	90	95	101	106	111	117	122	127	133
107 "	80	86	91	96	102	107	112	118	123	128	134
108 "	81	86	92	97	103	108	113	119	124	130	135
109 "	82	87	93	98	104	109	114	120	125	131	136
110 "	83	88	94	99	105	110	116	121	127	132	138
111 "	83	89	94	100	105	111	117	122	128	133	139
112 "	84	90	95	101	106	112	118	123	129	134	140
113 "	85	90	96	102	107	113	119	124	130	136	141
114 "	86	91	97	103	108	114	120	125	131	137	143
115 "	86	92	98	104	109	115	121	127	132	138	144
116 "	87	93	99	104	110	116	122	128	133	139	145
117 "	88	94	99	105	111	117	123	129	135	140	146
118 "	89	94	100	106	112	118	124	130	136	142	148
119 "	89	95	101	107	113	119	125	131	137	143	149
120 "	90	96	102	108	114	120	126	132	138	144	150
121 "	91	97	103	109	115	121	127	133	139	145	151
122 "	92	98	104	110	116	122	128	134	140	146	153
123 "	92	98	105	111	117	123	129	135	141	148	154
124 "	93	99	105	112	118	124	130	136	143	149	155
125 "	94	100	106	113	119	125	131	138	144	150	156
126 "	95	101	107	113	120	126	132	139	145	151	158
127 "	95	102	108	114	121	127	133	140	146	152	159
128 "	96	102	109	115	122	128	134	141	147	154	160
129 "	97	103	110	116	123	129	135	142	148	155	161
130 "	98	104	111	117	124	130	137	143	150	156	163
131 "	98	105	111	118	124	131	138	144	151	157	164
132 "	99	106	112	119	125	132	139	145	152	158	165
133 "	100	106	113	120	126	133	140	146	153	160	166
134 "	101	107	114	121	127	134	141	147	154	161	168
135 "	101	108	115	122	128	135	142	149	155	162	169
136 "	102	109	116	122	129	136	143	150	156	163	170
137 "	103	110	116	123	130	137	144	151	158	164	171
138 "	104	110	117	124	131	138	145	152	159	166	173
139 "	104	111	118	125	132	139	146	153	160	167	174
140 "	105	112	119	126	133	140	147	154	161	168	175
141 "	106	113	120	127	134	141	148	155	162	169	176
142 "	107	114	121	128	135	142	149	156	163	170	178
143 "	107	114	122	129	136	143	150	157	164	172	179
144 "	108	115	122	130	137	144	151	158	166	173	180
145 "	109	116	123	131	138	145	152	160	167	174	181
146 "	110	117	124	131	139	146	153	161	168	175	183
147 "	110	118	125	132	140	147	154	162	169	176	184
148 "	111	118	126	133	141	148	155	163	170	178	185
149 "	112	119	127	134	142	149	156	164	171	179	186
150 "	113	120	128	135	143	150	158	165	173	180	188
151 "	113	121	128	136	143	151	159	166	174	181	189
152 "	114	122	129	137	144	152	160	167	175	182	190
153 "	115	122	130	138	145	153	161	168	176	184	191
154 "	116	123	131	139	146	154	162	169	177	185	193
155 "	116	124	132	140	147	155	163	171	178	186	194
156 "	117	125	133	140	148	156	164	172	179	187	195
157 "	118	126	133	141	149	157	165	173	181	188	196
158 "	119	126	134	142	150	158	166	174	182	190	198
159 "	119	127	135	143	151	159	167	175	183	191	199
160 "	120	128	136	144	152	160	168	176	184	192	200
161 "	121	129	137	145	153	161	169	177	185	193	201
162 "	122	130	138	146	154	162	170	178	186	194	203
163 "	122	130	139	147	155	163	171	179	187	196	204
164 "	123	131	139	148	156	164	172	180	189	197	205

2.9 Tables for deriving the Ungerleider index using the cardiothoracic diameter, from the posteroanterior chest X-ray and body height and weight. The diagnosis of left ventricular hypertrophy is likely when the index is ≥10%, and this is supported further by electrocardiographic indices of left ventricular hypertrophy *(see below)*. From 'A study of the transverse diameter of the heart silhouette with prediction table based on the teleoroentgenogram' presented to the Association of Life Insurance Medical Directors of America by Dr Harry E. Ungerleider of the Equitable Life Assurance Society and Dr Charles P. Clark of the Mutual Beneficial Life Insurance Company (1938).

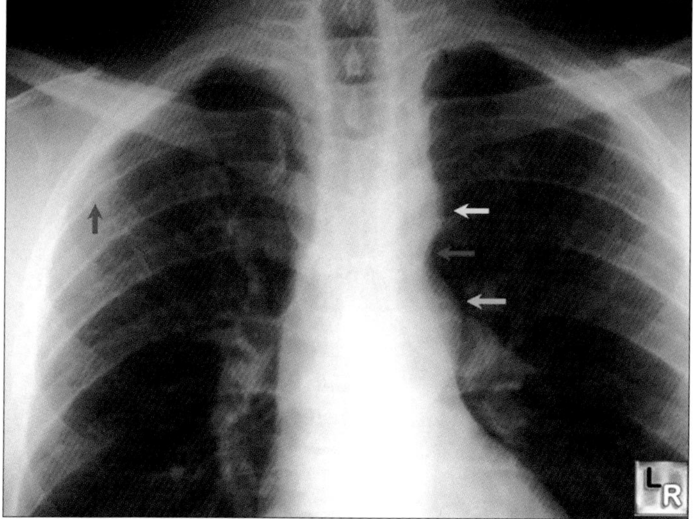

2.10 Chest X-ray demonstrating notching of the ribs in a patient with hypertension and aortic coarctation. Red arrows demonstrate the notching of the ribs and the two green arrows and blue arrows demonstrate the coarctation of the aorta. Post-stenotic widening of the aorta is indicated by the yellow arrow.

Electrocardiogram

The physician should be acutely aware of the necessity to diagnose LVH since it is a major independent risk factor. The electrocardiogram (ECG) is still the diagnostic procedure of choice and is of major value for the clinical diagnosis of LVH and other cardiac abnormalities. When LVH is demonstrated by ECG, there is little necessity for performing an echocardiogram (unless to recognize coexisting cardiac lesions or for assessing ventricular contractile function). On the other hand, the echocardiogram may be of particular value when there is no evidence of LVH by ECG, yet LVH is still suspected. As discussed in Chapter 1, the ECG indices of left atrial abnormality are the first signs of cardiac involvement from hypertension (*Table 2.16*) and provide evidence that the LVH has already adapted to its increased afterload by hypertrophy, a finding that is highly concordant with the fourth heart sound (atrial diastolic gallop rhythm or the *bruit de galop*). As hypertensive heart disease progresses further, LVH can be detected by other electrocardiographic criteria (*Tables 2.16, 2.17;* **2.11**).

Table 2.16 Abnormal diagnostic cardiac criteria*

Left atrial abnormality on ECG – two of four

- P wave in lead II ≥0.3 mV and ≥0.12 s
- Bipeak interval in notched P wave ≥0.04 s
- Ratio of P wave duration to PR segment ≥1.6 (lead II)

Left ventricular hypertrophy

- Ungerleider index ≥+15% on chest X-ray alone
- Ungerleider index ≥+10% on chest X-ray + two of the following ECG criteria:
  - – Sum of tallest R and deepest S wave ≥4.5 mV (precordial) (see *Table 2.17*).
  - – LV 'strain' – i.e. QRS and T wave vectors 180° apart (see 2.11)
  - – QRS frontal axis <0°
- All three ECG criteria (above)

ECG, electrocardiogram; LV, left ventricular.

*The reader is also referred to Figure 2.2.

Table 2.17 Accuracy of electrocardiographic QRS voltage criteria for left ventricular hypertrophy on autopsy

ECG criteria	*False negatives (%) (n)*	*False positives (%) (n)*	*Total false diagnosis (%)*
$R_1 + S_{I\,II}$ >2.5 mV	90 (275)	0.5 (172)	90.5
Greatest R + greatest S in V leads >4.5 mV	59 (92)	1.5 (62)	60.5
Greatest R + S in V leads >3.5 mV	65 (37)	6.0 (34)	71
$SV_1 + RV_5$ or RV_6 >3.5 mV	68 (275)	6.0 (172)	74
RV_5 or RV_6 >2.6 mV	77 (275)	4.0 (172)	81

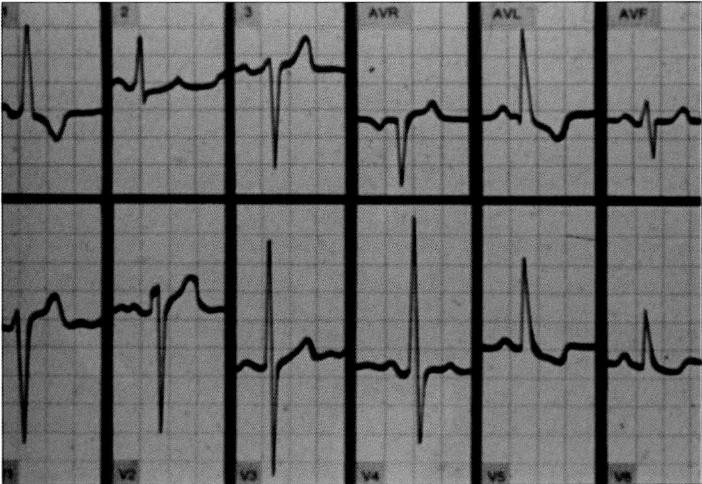

2.11 Electrocardiogram demonstrating left ventricular hypertrophy and strain in a patient with hypertension.

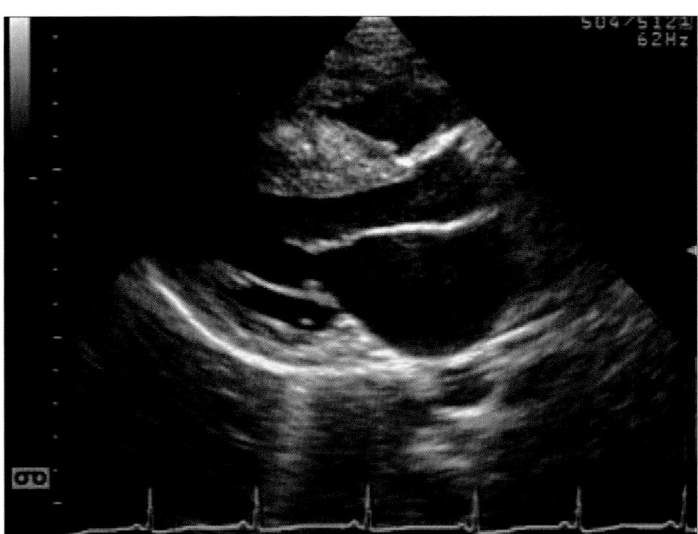

2.12 Echocardiogram.

Echocardiogram

The echocardiogram is a far more sensitive means for diagnosing LVH (**2.12**). Indeed, many patients with 'echo-LVH' may not yet have electrocardiographic evidence of LVH. However, it is important to appreciate that the echocardiographic diagnosis of LVH, even in its earliest stages, confers a significantly increased risk of premature cardiovascular morbidity and mortality that is independent of the height of either the systolic or diastolic pressure elevation. In addition to providing the structural evidence of increased LV mass and LV wall thickness (i.e. free wall and septum), this technique also provides important information concerning ventricular contractile and filling functions. Whereas the best methodology for assessing diastolic function may still be controversial, the E/A ratio has been of value for evaluating ventricular distensibility. Patients with atrial enlargement by ECG have true enlargement of that chamber, and this is associated with an impaired atrial emptying index on echocardiographic study that correlates with scintigraphic evidence of impaired ventricular filling. Furthermore, the existence of left atrial abnormality may be associated with an increased occurrence of atrial dysrhythmias. The echocardiogram is not indicated for every patient with hypertension; the ECG still remains more cost-effective. However, recent reports suggest that a limited echocardiogram (employing only M-mode indices) may be more cost-effective than the M-mode, 2D Doppler echocardiogram when only LVH is to be detected (*Table 2.18*).

Table 2.18 Indications for echocardiography in patients with hypertension

- To establish the existence of LVH when not demonstrated by ECG
- To evaluate the contractile function of the LV
- To assess the diastolic filling function of the LV
- To study the progression of cardiac involvement
- To investigate structural or function changes with treatment
- For research purposes
- For other clinical indications

ECG, electrocardiogram; LV(H), left ventricular (hypertrophy).

Other laboratory techniques

Although not indicated in all uncomplicated essential hypertensive patients (i.e. the largest subgroup of hypertensives), a number of tests are available to assess target organ effects of hypertension (*Table 2.19*).

Nuclear imaging

Myocardial scintigraphic scanning, using any of several nuclides, is of importance in assessing myocardial perfusion and cardiac function, particularly when myocardial ischaemia is of concern. Thus, in the patient with LVH associated with cardiac dysrhythmias or with treadmill abnormalities suggestive of ischaemic heart disease, the nuclear scan can be valuable. It is important to appreciate that a normal scan in a patient with hypertensive heart disease excludes neither the diagnosis of obstructive epicardial disease nor even the additional likelihood of small vessel arteriolar disease (e.g. 'silent ischaemia', 'microvascular angina'). Under these circumstances, the isotopic scan may not be adequate, and a better index of coronary flow reserve may be of value, using pharmacologically induced coronary vasodilation (e.g. with dipyridamole, adenosine). Other techniques to evaluate myocardial flow (and reserve) have included timed coronary inflow using radiocontrast material in flow and angiographic frame counts. Also under evaluation for their clinical applicability are magnetic resonance imaging and positron emission technology.

Intravenous urography

It is no longer necessary to perform routine intravenous urography (IVU) to evaluate every patient with essential hypertension. However, IVU is of value if there is a suggestion of coexisting renal disease, although selective renal arteriography is the study of choice if renal arterial disease is strongly suspected. It is also helpful to request that the radiologist obtain a post-arteriographic flat plate of the abdomen to determine whether the contrast material is excreted from the kidney and the renal sizes (i.e. lengths and widths of each kidney). The latter data should be tabulated in the patient's record to follow progression of disease with time. In general, the right kidney may be from 0.5 to 1.0 cm shorter than the left, so that if the left kidney is 0.5 to 1.0 cm shorter than the right there may be a greater likelihood of potential left renal arterial occlusive disease.

Table 2.19 Other laboratory investigations of value in the diagnostic evaluation of patients with hypertension

- Chest X-ray (PA and lateral projections)
- ECG (12-lead, conventional)
- Intravenous urogram ('hypertensive IVU')
- Renal arteriography
- Bilateral renal venous renin determinations
- Isotope renography and renal scans
- Thyroid function studies
- Plasma parahormone concentration
- Blood volume determination (plasma volume, RBC mass)
- Radioimmunoassay studies:
  - Plasma renin activity
  - Plasma angiotensin I or II or ACE concentrations
  - Human growth hormone concentration
  - Plasma insulin concentration
- Urinary hormone excretion studies (24-hour collection)
  - Catecholamine, VMA, metanephrine concentrations in urine
  - Plasma catecholamine concentration
  - Plasma aldosterone concentration
  - Corticosteroid and ketosteroid concentrations
  - Plasma atrial natriuretic peptide
- Clonidine suppression test for phaeochromocytoma (see Chapter 4)

Selective renal arteriography

If renal arterial disease is to be diagnosed, the renal arteries must be visualized. The significance of renal arterial disease has also been defined in terms of the renal pressor system (i.e. bilateral renal venous plasma renin activity). Thus, if the ratio of affected to unaffected kidney is 1.6 or more, there is further reason to ascribe significance to the existence of renal arterial lesion. Indications for intravenous urography and selective renal arteriography are presented in *Table 2.20*.

An additional consideration must be the pathological nature of the renal arterial lesion. The arteriographic findings provide considerable information to suggest not only the significance but also the natural history of the disease (see Chapter 5). For example, if the renal mass is severely contracted, the implication is that the lesion must be 'significant'. There are basically two types of renal arterial disease: the atherosclerotic and the nonatherosclerotic (or fibrosing) lesion. With respect to the former, hypertension may have preceded the development of the lesion (e.g. hypertension may facilitate the progression of atherosclerosis) or it may be the result of the arterial lesion (e.g. renovascular hypertension). Renal venous renin activity studies may provide useful information on the probable response to corrective surgery in patients with atherosclerotic plaques (and in patients with segmental lesions). Thus, if there is no evidence of increased production of renin by the 'affected' kidney, especially if the affected kidney is not contracted in size, it might be wiser to treat the patient pharmacologically and to follow that

Table 2.20 Specialized investigations of value in evaluating patients with hypertension suspected of having renal arterial disease

Investigation	*Indications*
Intravenous urography	• Consideration of renal parenchymal disease; history of frequent urinary tract infections, renal stones, obstructive uropathy; persistence of hypertension after toxaemia of pregnancy
Selective renal arteriography	• Abdominal, flank or back bruit (particularly with diastolic as well as systolic components); sudden onset of hypertension; sudden severity of pre-existing hypertension (i.e. loss of blood pressure control following adequate prior therapy)
	• Disparity in renal lengths (by urography or scintigraphy) of ≥11 mm
	• Assessment for renal transplantation
	• Renal venous renin activities: functional assessment of the arterial lesion(s) at the time of selective renal arteriography
	• Evaluation for progression of known renal arterial disease
	• Follow-up of previously diagnosed renal arterial disease (e.g. to assess reduction in renal size or to compare postoperative and preoperative studies)
	• Postoperative assessment for the patency of renal blood supply (i.e. in conjunction with digital subtraction arteriography)
	• Confirmation of suspected renal arterial disease of a patient allergic to radiocontrast material or concern for development of renal failure
Plasma renin activity	• Assessment for low-renin forms of hypertension (e.g. primary [peripheral venous blood] aldosteronism, volume-dependent hypertension)
	• Assessment of high-renin forms of hypertension (renal arterial disease or high-renin essential hypertension)

patient with periodic radiographic or isotopic studies (e.g. intravenous urography, renal scans or isotope renograms). If, on the other hand, renal parenchymal function seems to be deteriorating (as evidenced by further diminution of renal size or if the pressure becomes increasingly more difficult to control), surgical measures might be indicated. In any event, the physician should realize that atherosclerotic renal arterial disease is part of a much broader systemic vascular disease, and prior to any surgical procedure the patient should be evaluated for atherosclerotic vascular disease involving the coronary, cerebral, mesenteric and great vessels.

There are several types of the other form of renal arterial disease (i.e. fibrosing disease). Not infrequently, these patients present no family history of hypertension, but a renal arterial bruit may be audible over the abdomen or flanks. In these patients there is a higher probability that surgical correction of these lesions might be expected to be associated with a normalization of arterial pressures. In some of these patients, involvement of both renal arteries may be present; this is found most often with the 'string-of beads' type of lesion, also termed perimedial fibroplasia. Fortunately, this type of fibrosing lesion is one of the most common types and progresses relatively slowly, and the associated elevated blood pressure may be treated pharmacologically while the patient is periodically observed for evidence of progression of the arterial disease. Other types of fibrosing renal arterial disease are more likely to progress in severity. These types may be complicated by aneurysm formation, dissection and thrombosis of the renal artery. For these reasons, surgical treatment may be considered more urgent in these patients. However, the general physical condition of the patient should always be considered. For a more detailed discussion concerning the diagnosis, treatment and varieties of renal arterial disease and hypertension, the reader is referred to Chapter 7 and references therein.

Renal venous renin activity determinations

The importance of renal venous renin activity determinations in interpreting the significance of renal arterial disease has already been discussed, particularly in the patient with atherosclerotic and bilateral renal arterial disease. However, after many years of use, the author still has reservations that inability to demonstrate a specific ratio of renal venous renin activity means that surgical treatment will be unsuccessful. A sufficient number of patients with so-called 'normal' ratios have not been subjected to surgery to determine whether surgery has corrected the elevated arterial pressure. In addition, physicians have collected renin data differently; some patients have ceased pharmacological therapy prior to renal venous renin collections, and other patients have been treated with a stimulating dose of a diuretic, an ACE inhibitor or an angiotensin II (type 1) receptor blocker. At present, however, many authorities employ the captopril (25 mg or 50 mg) stimulation test. A positive test is one in which the plasma renin activity is at least 150% greater than the precaptopril administration level. To confuse this problem further, some patients continue to receive a variety of antihypertensive (and other) drugs that may suppress or stimulate plasma renin activity. It therefore seems valid to ask the following questions. First, how does premedication (for arteriography) affect the results? Second, how does prior introduction of radiocontrast material into the renal artery affect renin release, as contrast affects intrarenal haemodynamics? Third, if a patient is receiving antihypertensive therapy, how does this affect the release of renin by the affected and unaffected kidneys? Fourth, do the affected and unaffected kidneys respond similarly to the same doses of antihypertensive drugs, and how does this affect the release of renin by the affected and unaffected kidneys? Fifth, if these kidneys respond differently, what is the significance of the stimulation tests using low-sodium diet and diuretics of varying types? The answers to these questions are not yet complete; however, understanding of the problem has improved vastly in recent years.

Isotope renography and renal scans

The greatest value of these scans may be related to follow-up care of a patient with renal arterial disease once diagnosis has been made. Thus, if a renal arterial lesion has been demonstrated and the physician and patient elect to pursue pharmacological treatment or to observe for progression of disease, these non-invasive isotopic studies might provide evidence of further contraction of renal mass and delay in the renal appearance of the isotope. Isotopic renography has been utilized before and after oral administration of a single dose of captopril. The ACE inhibitor may help to assess potential participation of the lesion in reducing blood flow to the affected kidney.

Plasma renin activity

Without entering into the continuing controversy on the role of plasma renin activity (PRA) in current practice, a few words are indicated. First, the physician must be aware of the pitfalls in collection and the physiological implications of the results, and the drugs and physiological conditions that alter PRA (*Table 2.21*). Since PRA increases with intravascular volume contraction (see Chapter 1), it is not surprising that the patient with severely contracted intravascular volume (e.g. malignant hypertension) will have a high PRA and that the patient with volume-dependent hypertension (e.g. primary aldosteronism) will exhibit low PRA.

Table 2.21 Physiological and pharmacological factors that may affect plasma renin activity

- Upright posture +
- Time of day +/–
- Age –
- Menstrual cycle stage –
- Daily dietary sodium intake –
- Daily dietary ammonia intake +
- Diarrhoea +
- Vomiting +
- Neat blood donation +
- Diuretics +
- Vasodilators (direct acting smooth muscle) ACE inhibitors +
- ACE inhibitors +
- Oral contraceptive agents +
- Anaesthetic agents +
- Beta-adrenergic receptor inhibitors –
- Adrenergic inhibitors –

Hormonal studies

Radioimmunoassay technology has provided a means for diagnosis of a variety of hormonal types of hypertension (*Table 2.12*).

Ambulatory blood pressure monitoring

Another diagnostic technique (associated with some controversy) is that of 24-hour ambulatory sphygmomanometry. It is particularly useful when discrepancies exist between clinic and home blood pressure measurements and with cardiac findings related to height of pressure. Other situations that indicate usefulness might be related to nocturnal angina or 'spells' suggesting orthostatic hypotension (*Table 2.22*). In the final analysis, careful home blood pressure measurements and records using

Table 2.22 Indications for automated blood pressure recording

- To confirm blood pressure readings (e.g. clinic [white coat] hypertension)
- To determine variability of blood pressures during a 24-hour period
- To evaluate patients with systemic hypertension and 'spells' with suspected phaeochromocytoma, episodic hypertension, or similar diagnoses
- To evaluate hypotensive symptoms associated with antihypertensive medication or autonomic dysfunction
- To relate blood pressure elevation with episodes of angina pectoris or other cardiac symptoms
- To determine whether nocturnal angina is related to blood pressure elevation
- To evaluate carotid sinus syncope or pacemaker syndromes (together with Holter electrocardiographic monitoring)
- To provide confirmation that blood pressure is well controlled and that antihypertensive treatment is efficacious
- To evaluate antihypertensive drug resistance and 'repair'
- To determine whether blood pressure may be elevated when office blood pressures and whether associated target organ involvement (e.g. of heart, kidneys, and brain) is present
- To support insurance or other 'third party' needs, demonstrating control (or lack of control) of blood pressure
- For research purposes

instruments for self-measurement have been found to be useful and are cheaper. The author recommends the use of mercury sphygmomanometry (by another familial observer) or aneroid devices that are able to be calibrated and may be used by the patient. To this end, aneroid instruments with an attachable stethoscope to the cuff itself are extremely reliable and are easily purchased through local medical supply stores.

'White coat' hypertension

There is no doubt that blood pressure measurements obtained in the physician's office or other health care settings may be higher than pressures that are taken by the patient at home or in other relaxed settings as well as by automatic portable blood pressure measuring devices. For this reason, the author frequently instructs patients on how to take their own pressures at home, regularly at the same time using the same procedure, and report these pressures. These records are valuable in determining an effective treatment programme and in deciding whether the elevated pressure should be reduced with antihypertensive drugs. The author prefers the patient to use a mercury sphygmomanometer (usually employed by another family member) or an aneroid cuff in which the bulb and manometer are in a single entity that is attached to the cuff and can be held and inflated by the contralateral hand. These instruments can be calibrated, in contrast to electronic devices.

Patients with higher pressures in the clinic setting with 'normal' pressures at home are said to have 'white coat hypertension'; in these patients, home pressures are extremely useful. Some physicians also employ ambulatory and automatic devices which are, obviously, more costly and must be employed with some judgement. The validity of automatic versus clinic measurements is the subject of much debate. In the author's opinion, the 24-hour ambulatory pressures cannot define a truly normal pressure since, at present, there are inadequate normative data for individuals of all ages, both genders, and all races. Moreover, all epidemiological actuarial data are based on the 'casual' pressures that have been obtained in the clinic setting in millions of patients. Hence, the issue of whether the patient with 'white coat hypertension' is normal or 'hypertensive' remains to be defined. Until then, the author suggests that there are definite rules for the use of 24-hour (or less) ambulatory pressures, and these are presented in *Table 2.8*.

Further reading

Joint National Committee on detection, evaluation, and treatment of high blood pressure: the 1992 Report of the Joint National Committee on detection, evaluation, and treatment of high blood pressure (JNC-VI): *Arch. Intern. Med.* 1997;**157**:2413–2446.

Frohlich ED: Evaluation and management of the patient with essential hypertension. In: *Cardiology*. WW Parmley, K Chaterjee (eds). JB Lippincott, Philadelphia, 1994, pp.1–17. *These two papers present a more detailed discussion on the initial evaluation of the patient with hypertension.*

Oren S, Grossman E, Messerli FH, Frohlich ED: High blood pressure: side-effects of drugs, poisons, and food. *Cardiol. Clin.* 1988; **6**:467–474. *The reference presents a detailed discussion of the variety of agents that may exacerbate an elevation in arterial pressure, particularly in a patient with hypertension.*

Keith NM, Wagener HP, Barker NN: Some different types of essential hypertension: their course and prognosis. *Am. J. Med. Sci.* 1939;**197**:332. *The seminal article detailing the classification of hypertensive retinopathy.*

Wagener HP, Clay GE, Gipner JF: Classification of retinal lesions in presence of vascular hypertension: report submitted by committee. *Trans. Am. Ophthalmol. Soc.* 1947;**45**:57. *A different presentation of the graduations of severity of hypertensive retinopathy from the more specialized concept of the ophthalmologist.*

Chrysanthakopoulos SG, Frohlich ED, Adamopoulos PN, *et al.*: The pathophysiologic significance of 'stress polycythaemia' in essential hypertension. *Am. J. Cardiol.* 1976; **37**:1069–1072. *A discussion of the underlying mechanisms associated with polycythaemia in patients with hypertensive disease.*

Ungerleider HE, Clark CP: Study of the transverse diameter of the heart silhouette with prediction table based on the teleroentgenogram. *Am. Heart J.* 1939;**17**:92. *The original presentation of the relationship of chest X-ray evidence of left ventricular hypertrophy to anatomical evidence of cardiac enlargement in hypertension.*

Tarazi RC, Miller A, Frohlich ED, Dustan HP: Electrocardiographic changes reflecting left atrial abnormality in hypertension. *Circulation* 1966;**34**:818–822.

Messerli FH, Frohlich ED, Dreslinski GR, *et al.*: Serum uric acid in essential hypertension: an indicator of renal vascular involvement. *Ann. Intern. Med.* 1980; **93**:817–821.

Frohlich ED: Classic Papers Symposium: History of Medicine Series: Surrogate indexes of target organ involvement in hypertension. *Am. J. Med. Sci.* 1996;**312**:225–228.

Frohlich ED, Re RN: Pathophysiology of systemic arterial hypertension. In: *Hurst's The Heart*, 9th edn. RW Alexander, RC Schlant, V Fuster, RA O'Rourke, R Roberts, EH Sonnenblick (eds). McGraw-Hill Companies, New York, 1998, pp.1635–1650.

Hall DW: Diagnostic evaluation of the patient with systemic arterial hypertension. In: *Hurst's The Heart*, 9th edn. RW Alexander, RC Schlant, V Fuster, RA O'Rourke, R Roberts, EH Sonnenblick (eds). McGraw-Hill Companies, New York, 1998, pp.1651–1672. *The above five references provide the background for the surrogate indices of early target organ involvement of heart and kidney from hypertensive disease.*

Sheps SG, Frohlich ED: Limited echocardiography for hypertensive left ventricular hypertrophy. An opinion statement. *Hypertension* 1997;**29**:560–563. *This is the first paper to provide data and recommendations for clinical outcomes of echocardiography in patients with hypertension and for use of a more limited and cost-effective echocardiographic examination.*

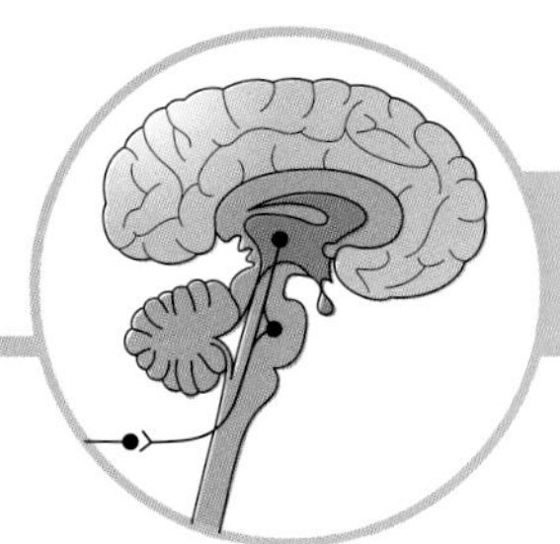

Chapter 3

Clinical pharmacology of antihypertensive agents

Introduction

In this chapter the available classes of antihypertensive agents will be discussed. The potential for individualized therapeutic approaches for specifically identified groups of patients is also considered, as well as for those with specific complications from hypertension or with associated cardiovascular risk factors. The evolution of the remarkable development of this large number of therapeutic options presents an exciting history and is a testimony to the major efforts of basic and clinical scientists from academia, industry and governments for over six decades (*Table 3.1*).

Lifestyle (non-pharmacological) interventions

The 3rd Joint National Committee report (and thereafter) included various non-pharmacological interventions for the treatment of hypertension for the first time. In these reports, several non-pharmacological modalities were included in considerable detail and, in subsequent reports, other interventions were added (*Table 3.2*). The more recent reports provide the evidence basis for inclusion of the non-pharmacological interventions; clearly, weight control and sodium restriction have the support of a large body of literature. The inclusion of alcohol moderation, a regular

Table 3.1 Major events in the development of antihypertensive therapy

1940: Thoracolumbar sympathectomy 1941: Rice diet 1950s: Drug therapy: • Ganglionic blocking agents • Reserpine • Hydralazine • Veratrium alkaloids • Thiazide diuretics • Guanethidine 1960s: Advances in therapy of secondary hypertensions: • Renal arteriography • Renal arterial surgery • Primary aldosteronism	More specific antiadrenergic therapy: • Methyldopa • Beta-adrenergic receptor inhibitors 1960–1972: Veterans Administrative Cooperative Study 1970s: Simplification of therapeutic concepts: • Screening • 'Stepped' care • Adherence Specific adrenergic receptors: • alpha-1 and alpha-2 receptors • beta-1 and beta-2 receptors	• Cardiospecificity • Intrinsic sympathomimetic activity Specialized vasodilators: • Arteriolar and venular dilation • Calcium antagonists 1980s: Renin–angiotensin system inhibition • Renin release • Large spectrum of controlled multicentre therapeutic trials • Angiotensin II receptor (type 1) blockers • Angiotensin-converting enzyme inhibitors

Table 3.2 Lifestyle modifications in the management of hypertension

Modification	*Recommendation*
Weight	Maintain normal body weight (BMI 18.5–24.9)
Dietary sodium	Reduce dietary sodium intake to no more than 100 mmol (mEq)/l (23 g sodium or 5.8 g sodium chloride)
Alcohol	Limit consumption to no more than two drinks per day (1 oz/30 ml of ethanol [e.g. 24 oz beer, 10 oz wine, or 3 oz 80% proof whisky]) in most men
Tobacco	Cessation as tobacco is a major cardiovascular risk and will interfere with hypertension control, especially with beta-blockers
Physical activity	Engage in regular aerobic (isotonic) physical activity such as brisk walking (at least 30 minutes per day, most days of the week)
Potassium	Eat a diet rich in fruits and vegetables

BMI, body mass index.

aerobic exercise programme, potassium supplementation and tobacco cessation is more recent. Smoking cessation has generally been emphasized in national and international guidelines for overall cardiovascular health value. However, it is of note that in the earlier Medical Research Council and Australian Mild Hypertension trials, one important finding was confirmed. Thus, if blood pressure was reduced by the same magnitude with diuretic or beta-adrenergic receptor blocker therapy in patients who smoked or did not, beta-blocker therapy failed to demonstrate protection against deaths from coronary heart disease and strokes in smokers.

Diuretics

Antihypertensive drugs have been available for over 50 years, and they continue to remain the mainstay of therapy. Inherent in their use is the rationale for low-sodium dietotherapy for reversing hypertensive disease and for enhancing the effectiveness of other antihypertensive agents. To be effective as the sole therapy (i.e. the Kempner rice–fruit diet), however, dietary sodium restriction must usually be <200 mg/day. It must be remembered that approximately one-half of dietary sodium intake is provided by sodium chloride; the other half is found in food additives and preservatives. Since this form of diet therapy is highly impractical, oral natriuretic agents which promote natriuresis and diuresis at all levels of the nephron (**3.1**) are used instead. There are three major classes of oral diuretic agents: thiazides and their congeners, 'loop' diuretics, and potassium-retaining agents.

Thiazides and congeners

These agents, including chlorothiazide, hydrochlorothiazide and a long list of their chemical congeners, are all similar in action, side-effects, and dosages (*Table 3.3*). To date, however, there have been no prospective, large-scale, double-blinded, controlled studies that have determined dose equivalencies, side-effects and end-points comparing any two agents. This statement is all the more pertinent since prospective studies comparing potency between chlorthalidone and a thiazide have not been reported.

However, one tablet of any one agent is considered to be equivalent to another compound in antihypertensive and natriuretic potency, as well as potential for hypokalaemic side-effects. According to the most recent joint national and international guidelines (i.e. JNC-V through JNC-VII and WHO/ISH), the thiazide diuretics (and their congeners) should be considered for initial therapy of patients with uncomplicated, essential hypertension, in contrast to the

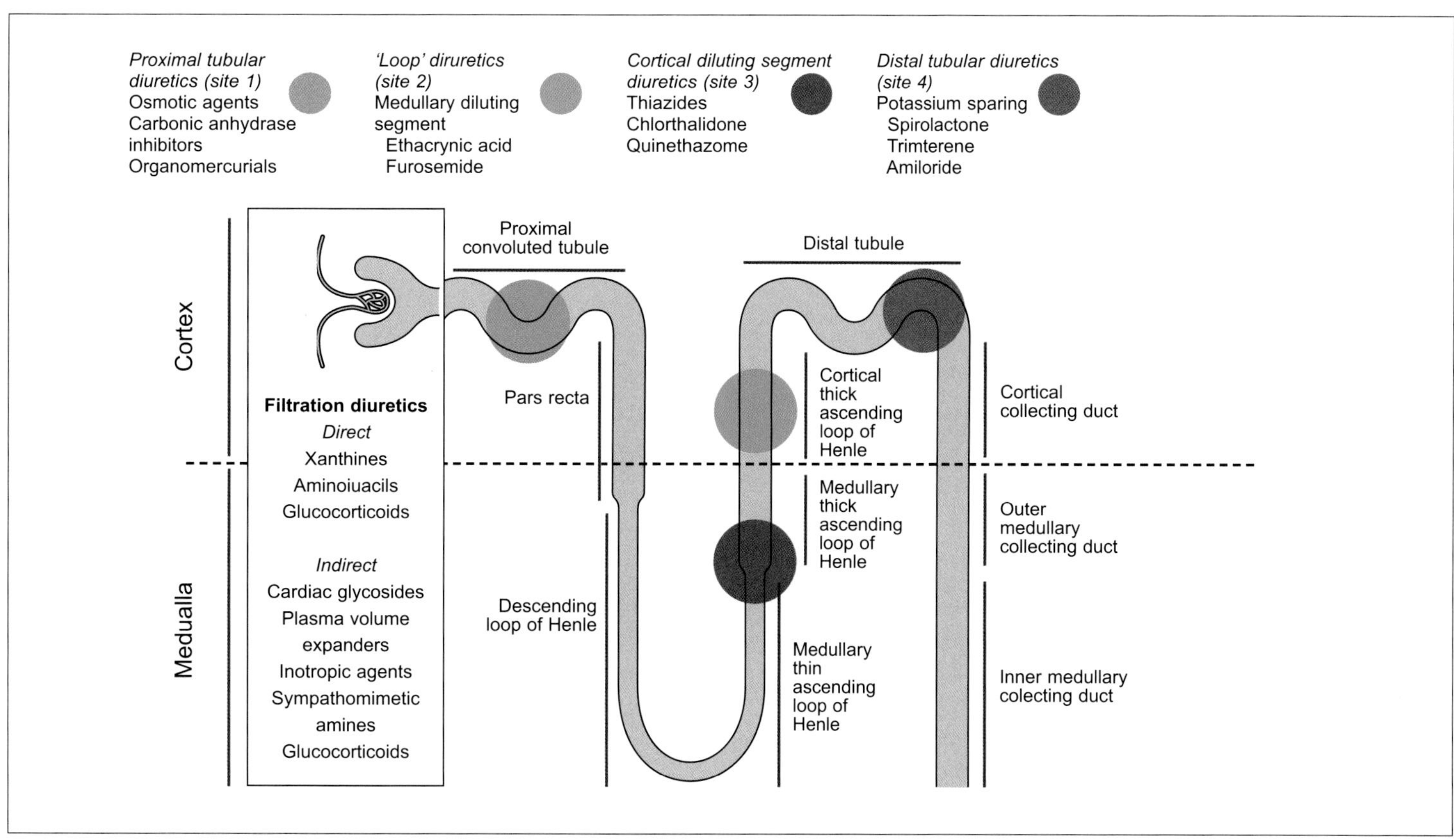

3.1 Sites of action on the nephron of the different classes of diuretic agents.

Table 3.3 Diuretic agents

	Agent	*Usual dose (mg/day)*
Thiazides	Chlorothiazide	125–500
	Chlorthalidone	12.5–25
	Hydrochlorothiazide	12.5–50
	Polythiazide	2–4
	Indapamide	1.25–25
	Metolazone	0.5–1.0
Loop	Bumetanide	0.5–2.0
	Furosemide	20–80
	Torsemide	25–10
Aldosterone antagonists	Eplerenone	50–100
	Spironolactone	25–50

'loop' diuretics. Thiazides are preferred unless the patient has previously demonstrated intolerance or idiosyncracy to these agents or unless renal excretory function is impaired. Increasing diuretic dosages (up to 1000 mg of chlorothiazide or 100 mg of hydrochlorothiazide) demonstrate increasing diuretic and associated metabolic effects. Larger doses offer little more natriuretic and diuretic efficacy but are more likely to enhance development of metabolic side-effects (e.g. hypokalaemia, hyperuricaemia) (*Table 3.4*). If, however, the patient has impaired renal excretory function, a loop diuretic may be prescribed in doses that may be progressively increased until, eventually, adequate diuresis is achieved (**3.2**).

It is important to recognize that the thiazides were originally prescribed in doses equivalent to ≥100 mg hydrochlorothiazide. This explains the greater likelihood for development of metabolic side-effects (*Table 3.4*) and the associated effects of higher doses. However, the more recent national and international guidelines have recommended an initial dose of 12.5–25 mg hydrochlorothiazide and 50 mg full dose, to provide therapeutic levels of thiazides at which the adverse side-effects are less pronounced.

Haemodynamics

The thiazides reduce arterial pressure initially as a consequence of contracted extracellular (plasma and interstitial) fluid volume but, later (after 6–10 weeks), as a consequence of reduced total peripheral resistance. Thus, following initial administration there is a decreased plasma volume and cardiac output that is associated with reduced total body sodium and water. Within a few days, arterial pressure falls (by 10–15%) associated with continued natriuresis and diuresis. After about 6 weeks, the plasma volume and cardiac output return towards pretreatment levels, and the reduced arterial pressure becomes associated with a decreased total peripheral resistance. The precise mechanism for the diminished vascular resistance remains incompletely understood (*Table 3.5*). It is likely that no one mechanism is responsible and all (or possibly still other unknown) mechanisms may participate in the overall antihypertensive action.

In addition to the hypotensive effect, there is an additional important consequence of attenuation of pressor agents and enhanced responsiveness to depressor sub-

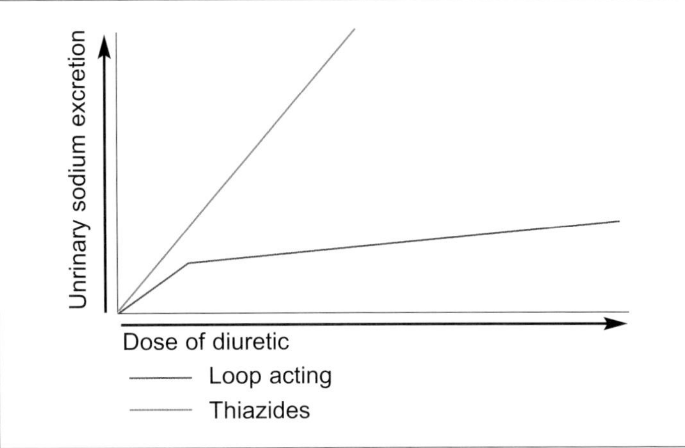

3.2 Dose–response curves of high ceiling ('loop') and thiazide diuretics.

Table 3.4 Metabolic effects of diuretic agents

- Hypokalaemia
- Hypomagnesaemia
- Hypercalcaemia
- Hyperuricaemia
- Hypercreatinaemia
- Carbohydrate intolerance
- Hyperlipidaemia

Table 3.5 Postulated mechanisms for diuretic-induced reduced vascular resistance

- Reduced 'waterlogging' in arterial wall
- Reversed autoregulation
- Altered transmembrane ionic potential across the vascular smooth muscle membrane
- Reduced responsiveness to endogenously generated neural stimuli and pressor substances
- Enhanced responsiveness to endogenously generated depressor substances or to antihypertensive agents
- Local action of generated prostacyclins
- Reduced release of renin from kidney
- Vasodilation via autocrine/paracrine mechanisms

stances. This latter effect provides the explanation for the antihypertensive synergism of diuretics with all other antihypertensive drugs except, possibly, calcium antagonists.

Mechanisms of action

The thiazide diuretics promote natriuresis through inhibition of carbonic anhydrase as well as active sodium reabsorption at the proximal and distal tubules. With natriuresis and volume contraction, the kidney releases renin from the juxtaglomerular apparatus, leading to the secondary generation of angiotensin II and consequent adrenal cortical release of aldosterone, thereby providing a feedback to the natriuretic stimulus. Additionally, potassium, magnesium and chloride ions are also lost in the urine, thereby inducing hypokalaemic alkalosis (i.e. secondary hyperaldosteronism) that may be confused with other causes of hypokalaemic alkalosis from hyperaldosteronism (e.g. primary aldosteronism, renal arterial disease, cardiac failure). Most notable with excessive dietary sodium intake, this secondary hyperaldosteronism can exacerbate diuretic-induced hypokalaemia by favouring sodium-for-potassium exchange at the distal tubule. Hence, one important means of reducing the hypokalaemia produced by thiazides is restriction of dietary sodium intake.

Metabolic effects

Hyperuricaemia

The thiazides increase tubular reabsorption of urate and plasma uric acid concentration. If this is severe enough, symptomatic gout may result. Therefore, if the uric acid concentration is borderline or elevated at the outset of therapy, or if there is a personal or family history of gout, uric acid should be rechecked intermittently during treatment anticipating potential gout. If uric acid concentrations exceed levels which can produce symptomatic gout, specific drug therapy may be prescribed to reduce serum uric acid concentration, e.g. the uricosuric agent probenecid or allopurinol, an inhibitor of the enzyme xanthine oxidase that reduces uric acid synthesis.

Hyperglycaemia

The thiazides may also induce carbohydrate intolerance or hyperglycaemia of varying degrees. When using the lower dose recommendations, the risk of development of diabetes requiring therapy may not be any greater than that with other antihypertensive drug classes (**3.3**). A number of underlying mechanisms of carbohydrate intolerance have been suggested (*Table 3.6*).

In the author's experience, overt insulin-dependent diabetes mellitus will not result from thiazide therapy de

Table 3.6 Potential diabetogenic mechanisms of thiazides

- Inhibition of pancreatic islet beta-cells
- Hypokalaemia
- Induction of 'end-organ' hyporesponsiveness or insensitivity to insulin
- Pre-existing carbohydrate intolerance exacerbated by the thiazide diuretic
- Coexisting diabetogenic factors: obesity, impairment of carbohydrate intolerance, hyperlipidaemia

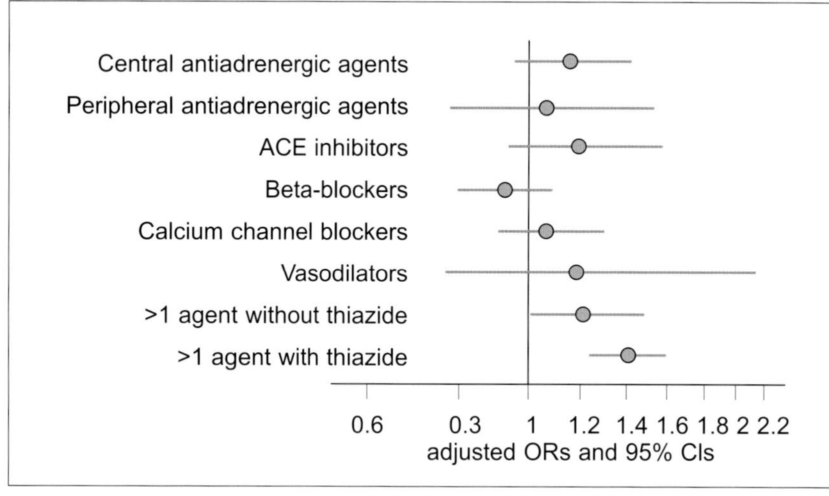

3.3 Risk of requiring hypoglycaemia therapy associated with the use of antihypertensive drugs, relative to the use of thiazides.

novo in hypertensive patients who do not already have abnormal carbohydrate intolerance prior to initiation of the diuretic. Should clinical diabetes mellitus exist or develop, this does not necessarily require discontinuance of the thiazide; it may be possible to prevent expression of diabetes with a lower dose (i.e. 12.5–50 mg hydrochlorothiazide) or by controlling the underlying problem with either dietotherapy and weight reduction alone, an oral hypoglycaemic agent or, if necessary, insulin. Alternatively, should this problem be of sufficient concern, another agent from a different antihypertensive drug class may be substituted for the initial diuretic.

Hypokalaemia

The problem of hypokalaemia had been minimized clinically in earlier years of thiazide therapy. However, it is now recognized that lower doses of thiazides provide similar control of pressure with less severe hypokalaemia and other metabolic side-effects. Furthermore, reduced dietary sodium intake (against a background of diuretic-induced secondary hyperaldosteronism) minimizes the hypokalaemic effect of the sodium-for-potassium distal tubular exchange mechanism. Addition of spironolactone, eplerenone or amiloride will augment the thiazide hypotensive effect although triamterene does not. However, each of these potassium-sparing agents protects against hypokalaemia (*Table 3.7*). The problem of sudden cardiac arrest has been clearly shown to be minimized by reducing the dose of thiazide or using potassium-sparing agents (**3.4**).

If primary hyperaldosteronism is considered to be the cause of this problem, the diuretic should be discontinued pending further clinical evaluation. Moreover, if the patient is receiving digitalis or there are other explanations for hypokalaemia (e.g. laxative abuse, chronic diarrhoea, vomiting, intestinal villous adenoma), the hypokalaemia should be corrected or an alternative antihypertensive agent should be considered. An angiotensin-converting enzyme (ACE) inhibitor (or an angiotensin II type 1 receptor antagonist) should be used with extreme caution in patients receiving potassium supplementation or any of the potassium-retaining agents, and in patients with impaired renal excretory function. In these patients, therapeutic

Table 3.7 Symptoms or complications of hypokalaemia

- Sudden cardiac death
- Cardiac dysrhythmias
- Polyuria
- Nocturia
- Muscle weakness
- Skin rash
- Suppression of bone marrow cellular elements

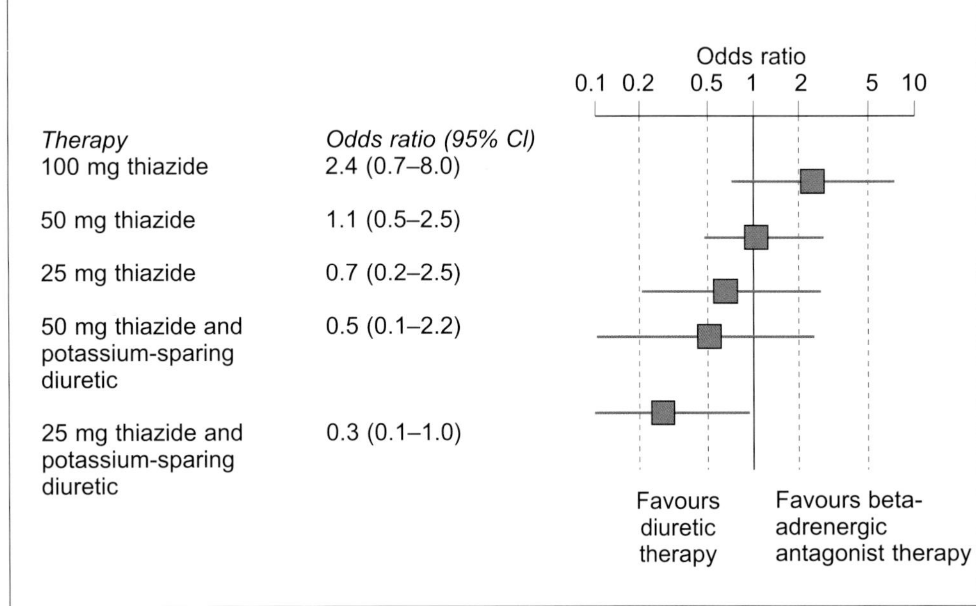

3.4 Risk of cardiac arrest with thiazides with and without potassium-sparing agents (compared with beta-blockers).

alternatives to diuretics should be considered. Although not diuretic agents, the calcium antagonists exert a natriuretic-like action (*Table 3.8*). Their 'natriuretic' action is mediated by a renal calcium-for-sodium exchange mechanism. This explains the symptom of increased nocturia associated with calcium antagonist therapy.

Loop diuretics

Bumetanide, ethacrynic acid and furosemide are the most potent loop-acting diuretic agents in clinical use. Unlike the thiazides, they promote natriuresis by inhibiting sodium transport at the ascending limb of the loop of Henle (**3.1**). Since more of the filtered sodium is delivered to the distal tubule for exchange, a greater degree of potassium wastage results. Their onset of action is more immediate, frequently within 20 minutes. Consequently, the diuresis is more rapid than the thiazides and their congeners produce, the rebound sodium and water retention may be more pronounced, and there may be greater potassium wastage. For these reasons, these compounds should be reserved for patients who cannot take the thiazides or when more prompt diuresis is desired, in patients with renal functional impairment or when an intravenous diuretic is necessary. In those patients with renal functional impairment, the dose–response curve of the loop agents is linear, unlike that of the thiazides (**3.2**). Thus, the 'loop diuretics' are not recommended for patients with uncomplicated, essential hypertension. In patients with secondary hyperaldosteronism (e.g. congestive heart failure), particular care should be exercised to prevent hypokalaemia and cardiac dysrhythmias. These patients present a very real potential for sudden cardiac death (**3.4**). One final important, but occasionally overlooked, indication for these agents is in the hypertensive patient who is already receiving antihypertensive drugs, including maximal thiazide doses. These patients may have developed pseudotolerance as a consequence of intravascular volume expansion, and this may be overcome by switching to the more potent loop-acting agent.

Table 3.8 Indications for use of a calcium antagonist in lieu of a diuretic

- Elderly – especially with isolated systolic hypertension
- Black race
- Renal parenchymal disease
- Steroid-dependent hypertension (e.g. primary aldosteronism, Cushing's disease or syndrome)
- History of metabolic side-effects from diuretics
- Volume-dependent essential hypertension
- Low plasma renin activity

Potassium-sparing agents

Spironolactone or eplerenone

These agents are discussed separately because they promote diuresis through a very specific mechanism: inhibition of the distal tubular action of aldosterone. Thus, by antagonizing the aldosterone-mediated sodium-for-potassium ion exchange mechanism, natriuresis and diuresis are effected without potassium wastage. Since much of the obligate sodium ion transport occurs at the level of the proximal tubule, the potency of these agents is not as great as that of thiazides. Nevertheless, they are particularly useful, either alone or in combination with a thiazide, for patients with primary and secondary hyperaldosteronism. Hence, in patients with hyperaldosteronism, the major value of these agents is that they achieve significant sodium and water excretion without depleting potassium (even when used with a thiazide).

Since spironolactone and eplerenone are effective in secondary hyperaldosteronism states, they may be of particular value in patients receiving digitalis (with cardiac failure) to correct or prevent that degree of hypokalaemia which may promote cardiac dysrhythmias. Since spironolactone (more than eplerenone) resembles progesterone in its chemical configuration, its side-effects may include gynaecomastia and mastodynia more frequently, a side-effect which may be more frequent (or noticeable) in men. This side-effect is claimed to be less frequent with the recently released compound eplerenone, which also antagonizes the renal action of aldosterone. The physician should also be aware of the potential for these agents to promote hyperkalaemia in patients with impaired renal function or if the patient is also receiving an ACE inhibitor or an angiotensin receptor blocker. This possibility should be of special importance in patients with chronic renal diseases or with cardiac failure; in these patients, supplemental potassium, with or without a potassium-sparing agent, should be used with extreme caution.

Amiloride and triamterene

These two agents are structurally related and they act upon the same non-aldosterone-dependent sodium-for-potassium renal tubular transport mechanism. Therefore, their action is entirely different from that of spironolactone or eplerenone. Both agents reduce arterial pressure when used with a thiazide to preserve potassium. However, although triamterene has an amiloride-like potassium-sparing action, it has minimal, if any, diuretic and antihypertensive properties. Moreover, as emphasized with spironolactone and eplerenone, these agents should be used with caution in patients with impaired renal function and, particularly, in patients receiving ACE inhibitors because of the potential for severe hyperkalaemia.

Adrenergic inhibitors

The present array of available sympatholytic compounds now makes it possible for the clinician to dissect pharmacologically many levels of the autonomic nervous system (**3.5**).

The first agents introduced were the ganglion-blocking drugs, drugs that selectively inhibit in the postganglionic neuronal terminal at the dorsal ganglia. Among the later agents introduced were those that deplete neurohumoral (i.e. norepinephrine [noradrenaline], serotonin [5HT]) agents from postganglionic nerve endings and in the adrenal glands and the central nervous system. Centrally acting agents stimulate alpha-adrenergic receptors in cardiovascular medullary centres (e.g. nucleus tractus solitarius) and reduce adrenergic outflow to the cardiovascular system and kidney and were introduced thereafter (*Table 3.9*).

Ganglion blockers

Cardiac autonomic inhibition attenuates cardiac reflexes. Hypotension results from reduced cardiac venous return to the heart, attenuation of reflexive increases in heart rate, and myocardial contractility. Other evidence of inhibited

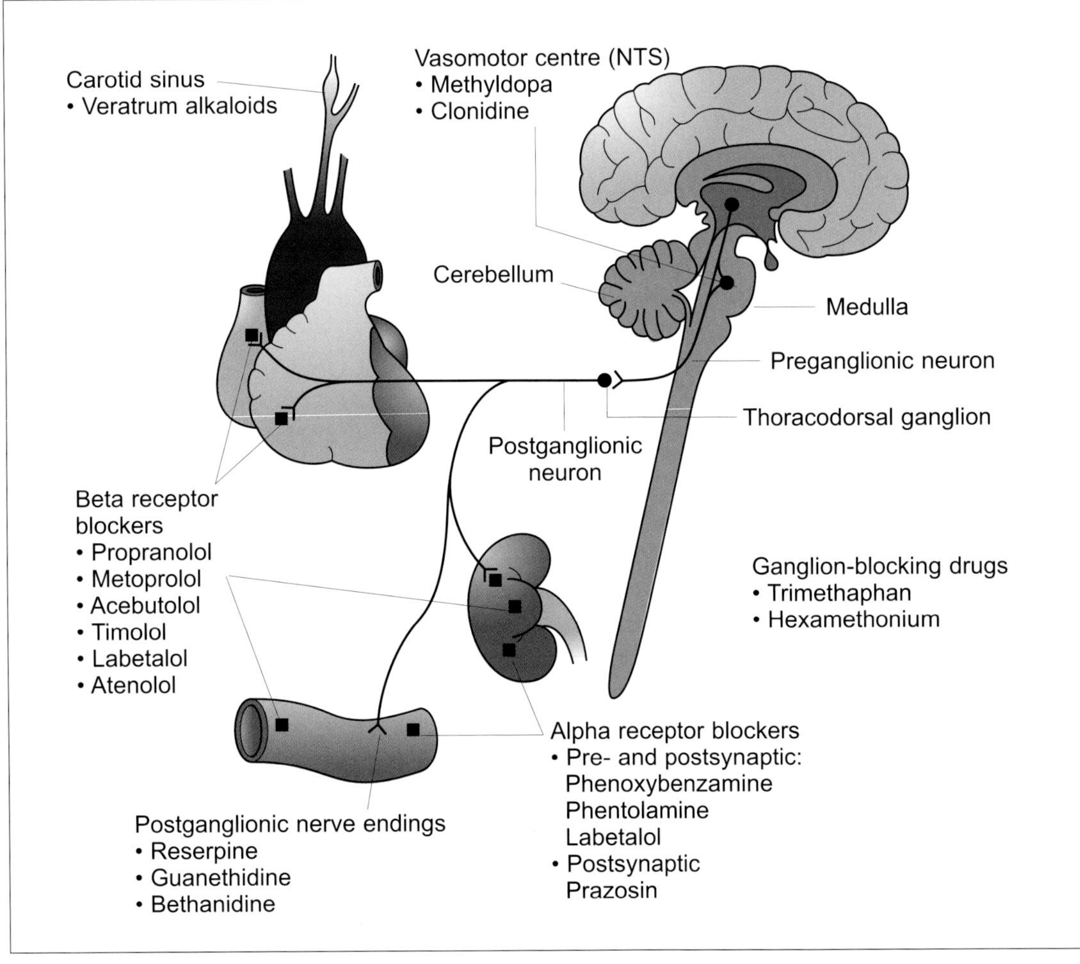

3.5 Sites of action of adrenergic blocking drugs.

Table 3.9 Sites of action of autonomic drugs

Level	*Stimulant*	*Inhibitor*
Cerebral-hypothalamic	Amphetamines	Barbiturates
		Antidepressants
Medulla	Pentylenemetrazol Ethamivan	Phenylthiazines
Ganglion	Tetraethylammonium Nicotine Dimethylphenylpiperazinium	Hexamethonium Pentolinium Trimethaphan
Adrenergic postganglionic neuron	Tyramine Ephedrine Cocaine	Reserpine Alpha-methyldopa Guanethidine Bethanidine
Alpha-adrenergic receptor site	Phenylephrine Methoxamine	Phentolamine Phenoxybenzamine
Beta-adrenergic receptor site	Isoproterenol	Propranolol Practolol

compensatory reflexes is shown by the abolition of the overshoot phase of the Valsalva manoeuvre, augmentation of postural hypotension, the 'tilt-back' overshoot of arterial pressure which occurs when the patient returns to the supine position, or postexercise hypotension. The former phenomenon is explained by the sudden return of pooled blood in the peripheral circulation; the latter is explained by the redistribution of circulating blood into the vasodilated skeletal musculature when the patient remains upright after exercise. The very same haemodynamic effects obtained with the ganglion blockers are also observed with postganglionic inhibitors (e.g. guanethidine), agents that deplete sympathetic nerve endings of norepinephrine (noradrenaline); however, in this situation the parasympathetic function which is observed with ganglion blockers is not inhibited.

Although ganglion blockers were the mainstay of treatment for severe hypertension many years ago, these agents are now used rarely, usually with intravenous formulation for immediate and controlled hypotension with certain severe hypertensive emergencies or for control of arterial pressure during certain operative (e.g. neurosurgical) procedures. In these circumstances, trimethaphan camsylate is infused intravenously (1 mg/ml) to produce instantaneous reduction of pressure; pressure immediately increases after dose reduction (or cessation). Antihypertensive effectiveness is enhanced during upright posture (i.e. by elevating the head of the bed) and with the concomitant use of diuretics or associated blood loss.

With these and all other adrenergic inhibiting (as well as the direct-acting smooth muscle vasodilating) agents, the phenomenon of pseudotolerance (intravascular volume expansion after control of pressure is achieved) will frequently occur unless a diuretic is administered. This explains why their hypotensive action is enhanced by diuretics. Since the ganglion-blocking drugs also inhibit parasympathetic nerve activity, intestinal and urinary bladder smooth muscle function is also inhibited, thereby predisposing to paralytic ileus and urinary retention. An additional side-effect (although not a complaint during intravenous infusion) is loss of penile erectile function.

Rauwolfia alkaloids

Included in this group are agents with varying potency and ability to deplete brain, adrenal glands and postganglionic sympathetic nerve endings of the biogenic amines (i.e. norepinephine [noradrenaline], epinephrine [adrenaline], dopamine, serotonin [5HT]). These compounds were used with greater frequency in the earlier years of antihypertensive drug therapy, and they are still used in many areas around the world. When administered by injection (e.g. reserpine, 1.0–5.0 mg), they are effective in treating patients with hypertensive emergencies or thyrotoxicosis. A test injection of 0.25 or 0.5 mg is worthwhile in order to avoid the excessive pressure reduction produced by larger doses. In recent years, with the advent of newer agents with less bothersome side-effects (e.g. reserpine-induced obtunded sensorium, depression), they are used rarely in hypertensive emergencies. However, when administered orally, they serve as mild antihypertensive compounds, although they must be used with a diuretic since when used alone their antihypertensive effect is minimal. They reduce arterial pressure through a fall in total peripheral resistance associated with a decreased heart rate and an unchanged cardiac output. Side-effects include nasal stuffiness relating to vasodilator action, postural hypotension, bradycardia, overriding parasympathetic gastrointestinal tract stimulation, mental depression and sexual dysfunction. The mental depression may be subtle and should be considered when evaluating any patient who has been receiving these agents over a prolonged time, particularly if there is any concern about behavioural changes.

Postganglionic neuronal depletors

Included among this class of drugs are guanethidine and guanadrel. The former compound has been available for patients with more severe hypertension for 50 years. The latter was introduced more recently for patients with less severe hypertension. Both compounds have similar actions; the lower doses used with guanadrel result in fewer side-effects. Guanethidine has a prolonged delay (up to 48 or 72 hours) in its hypotensive action which, once achieved, may persist for days or weeks (even as much as 1 month) after it has been discontinued. Both agents demonstrate haemodynamic effects similar to the ganglion blockers, although the additional parasympathetic inhibition is absent. There is a reduction in arteriolar resistance, peripheral venodilation with decreased cardiac venous return and cardiac output, attenuated cardiovascular reflexive adjustments, and reduced renal blood flow and (possibly) impaired renal excretory function. In the patient with adequate pretreatment renal functional reserve, the diminished renal excretory function may be expected to readjust itself. Additional side-effects include bradycardia, orthostatic hypotension, increased frequency of bowel movements (or diarrhoea from unopposed parasympathetic function) and retrograde ejaculation.

These adrenolytic compounds are taken up by the postganglionic nerve endings, thereby inhibiting norepinephrine (noradrenaline) reuptake. As a result, the postganglionic nerve endings become depleted. This concept is important since the commonly used tricyclic antidepressant drugs (e.g. imipramine, desipramine, amitriptyline and protriptyline) inhibit the nerve ending's ability to incorporate guanethidine and guanadrel. Thus, the antidepressants antagonize the antihypertensive actions of these drugs; conversely, when the antidepressant drug is discontinued, arterial pressure may fall suddenly and precipitously.

Centrally acting postsynaptic alpha-adrenergic agonists

Methyldopa has been used for over 45 years, and is still used widely in certain countries. Although originally thought to reduce arterial pressure through inhibition of the enzyme dopa-decarboxylase, its action was later postulated to work by false neurotransmission. This action implies conversion of the drug alpha-methyldopa to its less biologically active amine alpha-methylnorepinephrine which, in turn, binds to peripheral alpha-adrenergic receptor sites in competition with endogenous norepinephrine (noradrenaline). However, its action has recently been shown to be mediated through its false neurohumoral substance, alpha-methylnorepinephrine in brain. The false neurotransmitter stimulates postsynaptic alpha-adrenergic receptor sites in brain (i.e. nucleus tracti solitarii), thereby resulting in reduced adrenergic outflow from the medullary centres to the cardiovascular system and kidney. This is achieved haemodynamically through a reduced arteriolar resistance with a lesser fall in venous tone than with the agents described above. Consequently, cardiac output and renal blood flow are not reduced as much and, therefore, postural hypotension is less commonly observed with these agents.

The most common side-effects of these drugs include dry mouth, lethargy, easy fatiguability, somnolence and sexual dysfunction. These effects may be attributed to the central action of methyldopa and disappear shortly after therapy is discontinued. Less common side-effects include Coombs' test-positive reactions, haemolytic anaemia, high fever after initial treatment, and hepatotoxicity; all remit on withdrawal of therapy.

Clonidine, guanabenz and guanfacine although chemically different from methyldopa share certain pharmacological actions. They reduce arterial pressure primarily through a decreased vascular resistance as a result of central stimulation of alpha-adrenergic receptor sites in the nuclei tracti solitarii. The reduced adrenergic outflow from brain also inhibits renal renin release.

Occasionally, when there is the possibility of a phaeochromocytoma, the differential diagnosis may be difficult. The patient may have many symptoms that are suggestive of the adrenal catecholamine-producing tumour and measurement of circulating catecholamine levels is indicated. Normal blood concentration of norepinephrine (noradrenaline) is usually <100 pg/ml and concentrations in patients with phaeochromocytoma usually exceed 600 pg/ml. Since it is not usually possible to suppress catecholamine levels resulting from a phaeochromocytoma and there may be some question in those patients with intermediary levels (between 100 and 600 pg/ml), the clonidine suppression test may be of value. Clonidine is administered in three successive hourly doses of 0.1 mg; the pretest elevated catecholamine level is reduced to normal levels in patients who do not have the adrenal tumour. Patients with essential hypertension and borderline elevated levels of norepinephrine (noradrenaline) as well as patients with idiopathic mitral valve prolapse will demonstrate suppression of the elevated levels.

These agents share many side-effects of the other adrenergic inhibiting compounds. One more common side-effect associated with clonidine is the possibility of a precipitous rebound of arterial pressure after abrupt withdrawal of the drug. When this occurs, symptoms of palpitations and tachycardia can be treated with a beta-adrenergic blocking drug, and the pressor phenomenon can be counteracted by injection of an alpha-adrenergic blocking drug (e.g. phentolamine) and/or reinstitution of the clonidine or another adrenergic inhibitor or another antihypertensive agent. Clonidine has been made available more recently as a transdermal patch (long-acting) medication that apparently has made these rebound episodes less likely.

Pre- and postsynaptic (alpha-1 and alpha-2) receptor antagonists

The earliest developed alpha-1 and alpha-2 receptor blocking drugs such as dibenzylene have limited usefulness today. They continue to be used (e.g. phentolamine 5–10 mg intravenously) for unexplained pressor episodes that suggest excessive release of catecholamines. Since pargyline hydrochloride and other monoamine oxidase inhibitors are still available for hypertension or, more frequently, as antidepressant agents, they also may provoke a hypertensive crisis after ingestion of certain foodstuffs (e.g. Chianti wine, marinated foods, certain cheeses) containing tyramine. The alpha-adrenergic blocking compounds are valuable in treating these pressor crises because the tyramine contained in these foods releases stored norepinephrine (noradrenaline) from the nerve endings, which when released is less able to be degraded in the presence of monoamine oxidase inhibitors.

Postsynaptic (peripheral) alpha receptor antagonists

There are two types of alpha-adrenergic receptors in the periphery. When the postsynaptic alpha-adrenergic receptors are stimulated by catecholamines released from the postganglionic nerve ending, arteriolar and venular constriction result. When presynaptic alpha-2 receptors are stimulated, further release of the norepinephrine (noradrenaline) from the nerve ending into the synaptic cleft is inhibited. Thus, in contradistinction to the alpha-1 and alpha-2 receptor-inhibiting compounds discussed above (i.e. phentolamine and phenoxybenzamine), those agents that selectively block the postsynaptic alpha-1 receptors (doxazosin, prazosin and terazosin) do not prevent alpha-2 receptor stimulation. Haemodynamically, the alpha-1 adrenergic receptor antagonists reduce arterial pressure as a result of reduced total peripheral resistance (without associated reflexively increased heart rate, cardiac output or myocardial contractility). They may produce postural hypotension, often after the first dose is administered. Consequently, treatment is initiated usually with the lowest dose, taken at bedtime and with cautionary advice to assume upright posture slowly during the night. This advice is particularly valuable for the man with benign prostatic hyperplasia who takes this medication at bedtime. With more prolonged treatment, higher doses may be required. Intravascular volume expansion may occur with this adrenergic inhibitor, and will be associated with 'pseudotolerance.' Pseudotolerance can be offset by the addition of a diuretic; however, this may exacerbate the potential for postural hypotension. The volume expansion without an added diuretic may be associated with oedema and, perhaps, shortness of breath suggesting the possibility of cardiac failure. This problem occurred frequently enough during the ALLHAT multicentre trial, leading to the discontinuance of doxycycline from the study. A newer alpha-1A receptor inhibitor has been introduced (tamsalosin) which minimally reduces arterial pressure, but acts to relax prostatic smooth muscle cells, thereby ameliorating symptoms without unwarranted blood pressure reduction.

Beta-adrenergic receptor blocking agents

The beta-adrenergic receptor blocking drugs have been considered important alternative agents for the initial treatment of hypertension for over 40 years. These agents inhibit stimulation of cardiovascular beta-adrenergic receptor sites by adrenergic neurohumoral substances (e.g. norepinephrine [noradrenaline], epinephrine [adrenaline]) released from the postganglionic nerve ending or adrenal medulla. By inhibiting beta-receptor stimulation, their effects of increased peripheral resistance, heart rate, myocardial contractility and myocardial metabolism may be minimized. Moreover, because renal beta-adrenergic receptor sites in the juxtaglomerular apparatus are also inhibited, renal renin release is reduced.

Haemodynamics

The decreased arterial pressure is associated with a reduced cardiac output, although (the calculated) total peripheral resistance increases. Heart rate, myocardial tension and contractility, and myocardial metabolism are also inhibited. The reduced cardiac output (often by 20–25%) may not be associated with proportionate flow reductions in every organ. In fact, renal blood flow and excretory function may not diminish at all with beta-blocking therapy since the reduction in organ blood flows depends upon the number and affinity of beta-adrenergic receptor sites in each of the organ circulations. Thus, even though arterial pressure reduction is associated with reduced cardiac output and increased total peripheral resistance, effects on the heart and kidney may not be as detrimental as assumed. Myocardial oxygen demand is reduced and renal blood flow may remain unchanged or even increased as renal vascular resistance diminishes. In contrast, skeletal muscle and splanchnic organ blood flows are reduced. The reduced skeletal muscle blood flow may explain the fatigue experienced during exercise by some patients. Another important feature of these agents is the lack of expansion of intravascular volume as arterial pressure declines. Nevertheless, the diuretics will augment the antihypertensive effectiveness of the beta-blocking drugs; hence, they are frequently prescribed in combination.

At present, many beta-blocking agents are available for antihypertensive therapy; carvedilol and labetalol possess in a single molecule both alpha- and beta-adrenergic receptor inhibiting properties. Six agents (acebutolol, betaxolol, bisoprolol, carteolol, penbutolol and pindolol) possess cardiostimulatory (intrinsic sympathomimetic activity, ISA) properties and, hence, these agents may not reduce heart rate and cardiac output as much as those agents without ISA. They may, therefore, be of value in patients with pre-existing bradycardia or low cardiac output syndromes. It is important to know that those agents possessing ISA should not be used for the secondary prevention of cardiac death following myocardial infarction. The cardioselective beta-blockers (acebutolol, atenolol, celiprolol, metoprolol) probably exceed this property in the doses prescribed for the treatment of hypertension and angina pectoris, and are as effective as the non-cardioselective agents nadolol, propranolol and timolol. Nevertheless, the cardioselective agents may have value for patients who live in colder climates and who have symptoms of Raynaud's phenomenon or peripheral arterial insufficiency in winter months. The beta-blocking agents have therefore been found to be of particular value for the initial treatment of specific patients with hypertension (*Table 3.10*).

However, due to the systemic inhibition of beta-adrenergic receptors, this form of initial antihypertensive therapy should not be used under several circumstances (*Table 3.11*). In recent years, the beta-blockers have been advocated for patients with cardiac failure. Particular care must be taken in order not to exacerbate the condition, particularly in patients with severe hypertensive heart disease. Unfortunately, few patients with hypertension have been included in the multicentre trials evaluating beta-blockers for cardiac failure. Notwithstanding this cautionary note, some new beta-blocking compounds with beta-1 receptor vasodilator agonism and beta-2 cardiac muscle antagonism have been approved (e.g. carvedilol) for treatment of specific patients with cardiac failure, and the

Table 3.10 Indications for beta-adrenergic receptor antagonists

- Hyperdynamic beta-adrenergic circulatory state
- Other hyperkinetic circulatory states (i.e. with faster heart rate, symptoms of cardiac awareness, palpitations related to enhanced myocardial contractility)
- White race (when used alone) – all racial groups are similar when thiazide is added to the beta-blocker
- Previous myocardial infarction
- Cardiac dysrhythmias responsive to beta-blockers (e.g. catecholamines)
- Idiopathic mitral prolapse syndrome
- Already taking a beta-blocker in lower doses than for hypertension (e.g. for migraine, muscle tremor, glaucoma)

Table 3.11 Indications for withholding (or using with caution) beta-adrenergic inhibiting agents

- History of asthma
- Symptomatic chronic obstructive lung disease
- Heart block of second degree or more
- Severe peripheral arterial insufficiency
- Depression, hallucinations, nightmares (or vivid dreams)

preliminary results look promising. Another beta-blocker (sotalol) has been useful for certain cardiac dysrhythmias.

If full doses of the selected beta-blocking agent fail to control arterial pressure, the addition of a diuretic (or agents belonging to other classes) may be effective, particularly in the patient with coronary artery disease (e.g. a dihydropyridine calcium antagonist). However, caution should be exercised in the latter circumstance, since the negative and chronotropic effects of some calcium antagonists (e.g. non-dihydropyridines) may exacerbate the effects already provided by the beta-blocking agents.

Finally, negative statements have been made concerning the use of beta-blocking drugs in patients with diabetes mellitus. If that patient is taking insulin, it is true that the beta-blocker may mask the cardiovascular symptoms associated with catecholamine excess (e.g. episodes of hyperinsulinism). However, in general, studies have repeatedly demonstrated that long-term survival is improved with beta-blockers in both diabetic as well as non-diabetic patients (*Table 3.10*).

Direct-acting smooth muscle vasodilators

When beta-adrenergic blocking therapy was introduced there was a resurgence of interest in direct-acting smooth muscle vasodilating drugs for hypertension. These agents had been used with varying success in patients with cardiac failure. Hydralazine and minoxidil act by decreasing arteriolar resistance; but, with the fall in total peripheral resistance and arterial pressure, there is reflex cardiac stimulation unless offset by an adrenergic inhibitor (e.g. beta-blocker). For this reason, these agents should be used with caution in hypertensive patients with myocardial infarction, angina pectoris, cardiac failure or dissecting aortic aneurysm, because the reflexive cardiac effects of increased heart rate, cardiac output, myocardial contractility, and the rate of aortic blood flow will exacerbate these underlying cardiac conditions. Other side-effects include headache and nasal stuffiness, attributable to local vasodilation and fluid retention and oedema (i.e. pseudotolerance), which occurs more frequently with minoxidil. One unique side-effect of hydralazine is precipitation of a lupus erythematosus-like syndrome, which occurs more frequently in patients receiving more than 400 mg/day. A common side-effect from minoxidil is hirsutism, which is particularly unwanted by women. When hydralazine is administered by injection (10–15 mg intravenously), there is a prompt reduction in pressure.

Another parenteral direct-acting smooth muscle vasoclilator, diazoxide, is a non-natriuretic thiazide congener that must be injected rapidly (in a single bolus dose of 300 mg or in successive pulsed bolus divided doses) in order to prevent intravascular binding with circulating albumin. Diazoxide also should not be administered to the hypertensive patient with cardiac failure, angina pectoris, myocardial infarction, or an actively dissecting aortic aneurysm, for the reasons described above. It is, however, of value for the patient with acute hypertensive encephalopathy, intracranial haemorrhage and severe malignant or accelerated hypertension (without cardiac failure), in whom rapid and immediate reduction in arterial pressure is mandatory.

Sodium nitroprusside, an intravenous vasodilator, is very useful in hypertensive emergencies. This agent, infused by microdrip (60 mg/ml), instantly reduces arterial pressure; as the infusion rate is decreased, pressure rapidly returns to pretreatment levels. Since the agent reduces cardiac preload by venular (as well as arteriolar) dilation, it produces less cardiac venous return without an increase in heart rate or cardiac output. The drug therefore has particular value in treating severely hypertensive patients with myocardial infarction, cardiac failure (even with acute pulmonary oedema) or dissecting aneurysm. The drug is metabolized to thiocyanate, which may produce thiocyanate toxicity with prolonged infusion. Hence, monitoring of blood thiocyanate levels in these severely ill patients is important.

Angiotensin-converting enzyme inhibitors

This class of antihypertensive agents is also effective as monotherapy for patients with hypertension of all degrees of severity, including refractory hypertension, and patients with left ventricular hypertrophy, angina pectoris and cardiac failure. They reduce arterial pressure by inhibiting the generation of the haemodynamically active octapeptide angiotensin II from the inactive decapeptide angiotensin I (**3.6**). Inhibition of angiotensin-converting enzyme (ACE), therefore, reduces the generation of angiotensin II as well as the degradation or inactivation of the naturally occurring, potent vasodilator bradykinin. Furthermore, since angiotensin II interacts with the neurohormone norepinephrine (noradrenaline) in certain brain centres and peripheral nerve endings, less angiotensin II may be available for its central neural action. This may explain why reflexive cardiac stimulation is not generally recognized with these agents. Several investigators have suggested that there is also an increased availability of prostacyclin with ACE inhibition, and that the role of increased circulating kinins may be important in the overall antihypertensive action. Bradykinin and angiotensin II also appear to have opposite effects in the endothelial cell: bradykinin stimulates production of the local endothelial vasodilating agent nitric oxide (NO), whereas angiotensin II reduces NO. Recent studies have demonstrated that the entire renin–angiotensin system (with the possible exception of renin itself) exists in the vascular wall and in the cardiac myocyte (**3.6**). These findings provide an important mechanism favouring the effectiveness of ACE inhibitors in patients with normal and low plasma renin activity and, perhaps, even in patients following nephrectomy.

Haemodynamically, these agents reduce arterial pressure as a result of arteriolar dilation and a reduced total peripheral resistance, and heart rate and cardiac output do not increase reflexively. Renal blood flow usually increases in association with the reduced renal vascular resistance. Since glomerular filtration rate usually remains stable, the renal filtration fraction diminishes, suggesting that the reduced glomerular hydrostatic pressure results from efferent as well as afferent glomerular arteriolar dilation. These effects provide the mechanism for the value of ACE inhibitors in patients with proteinuria associated with end-stage renal disease with hypertension or diabetes mellitus.

ACE inhibitors are effective in patients with low and normal plasma renin activity as well as in patients with renin-dependent forms of hypertension. In this regard, they have great value in hypertensive patients with unilateral renal arterial disease with one normally functioning kidney, congestive heart failure or high-renin essential hypertension. They are useful as monotherapeutic agents, and their effectiveness is enhanced by an added diuretic. Reports have also suggested their effectiveness when employed with calcium antagonists. Moreover, these agents promote arteriolar dilation via their endothelial action and it has also been shown that they prevent development of cardiac failure through ventricular remodelling when given following myocardial infarction. This effect appears to occur by preventing the mitogenic effect of angiotensin in promoting fibrosis in the ventricular extracellular area as well as apoptosis in the entire wall itself.

A large number of ACE inhibitors are available: benazepril, captopril, enalapril, lisinopril, moexipril, quinapril, ramipril and trandolapril. Although there may be important pharmacodynamic and pharmacokinetic differences or even in their effects on the local tissue renin–angiotensin system, these drugs are nevertheless quite similar in their overall clinical effects, suggesting a class effect.

The ACE inhibitors have a remarkably low incidence of side-effects. This is in contrast to the earlier reports with captopril that suggested mandatory monitoring for leukopenia and proteinuria during the first few months of therapy. Since then, long-term studies which included patients with less severe and less complicated forms of hypertension have indicated that those effects occurred more frequently in patients with impaired renal function prior to therapy or in those who were receiving immunosuppressive therapy. Angioneurotic oedema following ACE inhibitors is an absolute contraindication for ACE inhibitors; likewise, they are strictly contraindicated in pregnancy, in patients with unilateral renal arterial disease in a solitary kidney, or in patients with bilateral renal arterial disease. Moreover, these agents should be used with extreme caution in conjunction with supplemental potassium therapy (or with potassium-retaining agents) since severe hyperkalaemia may result as a consequence of reduced aldosterone.

Other side-effects associated with ACE inhibitors include rash and cough, which disappear following cessation of therapy. The dry, unproductive cough may occur in approximately 8–13% of patients, and can occur with all the ACE inhibitors. Not all patients with this side-effect feel that it is sufficiently bothersome to warrant discontinuation of therapy. If the drug is discontinued, the cough will probably recur when the patient is rechallenged with the same or another ACE inhibitor. If the blood pressure response is successful with an ACE inhibitor, it may be useful to replace the ACE inhibitor with an angiotensin II receptor antagonist in patients with cough. Although the mechanism underlying cough has not been explained conclusively, it is likely to be on the basis of increased kinins resulting from inhibition of kinin degradation, and the effect of kinins on the pulmonary receptors that initiate cough. Since angiotensin II antagonists act by competitive antagonism at the receptor level and not by action on ACE, they do not affect kinin degradation and therefore do not produce cough.

Angiotensin II receptor antagonists

Angiotensin II exerts its action on vascular smooth muscle, heart, kidney, adrenal cortex, brain and other end-organs through angiotensin II (type 1) receptor stimulation (**3.6**). Several types of angiotensin II receptors have been identified, and specific type 1 (AT-1) receptor antagonists have been synthesized (candesartan, eprosartan, losartan, irbesartan, tasosartan, telmisartan, valsartan). These agents are active when taken orally. Antagonism of angiotensin II (type 1) receptors attenuates the actions of angiotensin II in the heart and vessel wall generated by incomplete ACE inhibition or by the enzyme chymase (primarily in heart). As with other agents that inhibit the renin–angiotensin system, the effects of angiotensin II receptor antagonists are markedly enhanced by a diuretic.

In those patients who respond to these drugs, the pressure reduction is mediated though a fall in total peripheral resistance; heart rate, cardiac output and myocardial contractility are not increased reflexively in response to the pressure reduction. Recent multicentre studies have demonstrated that these agents reduce efferent as well as afferent glomerular arteriolar resistance with associated reduction in glomerular hydrostatic pressure similar to the effects of ACE inhibition. These agents also reduce left ventricular mass and cardiac failure following myocardial infarction. As a consequence of these multicentre trials, these agents have been shown to prevent progression of end-stage renal disease in hypertension and diabetes, as well as stroke and cardiac failure following myocardial infarction.

Renin inhibitors

At the time of writing, only one pharmacological agent (aliskiren; US tradename Tekturna) that directly inhibits the rate-limiting biochemical step by impairing the action of renin to promote the conversion of angiotensinogen to angiotensin I. As a result, the cascading conse-quences of the renin–angiotensin–aldosterone system are markedly inhibited. The clinical experiences of this new compound are just becoming available, but the following information seems established. The drug reduces arterial pressure in a dose-dependent fashion, suppresses plasma renin activity in combination with a diuretic, is approved for once-daily oral administration, and the agent is clinically safe and effective when used alone as well as with other antihypertensive agents (e.g. a diuretic, calcium antagonist, ACE inhibitor, an ARB). To date, there have been no major adverse effects and, because it has no action on angiotensin-converting enzyme, treatment is not associated with cough, but angioneurotic oedema remains a caution and hyperkalaemia is still possible if this agent is used with an ACE inhibitor or an ARB. Thus, this agent will be useful in the treatment of patients with essential hypertension and there is great promise for patients with renal functional impairment because of its antiproteinuric effects experimentally.

Calcium antagonists

Calcium antagonists have been available for almost 50 years and form, without a doubt, the most heterogeneous of all antihypertensive drug classes in chemical structure, mode of action and clinical indications. Nevertheless, they have a certain commonality of action physiologically: inhibition of the availability of calcium ions in cardiac and vascular smooth muscle cells, thereby inhibiting the myocyte contractility and reducing heart rate (particularly the non-dihydropyridine compounds). At least four receptors to calcium channels have been cloned, each being responsive to calcium antagonist inhibition. This may explain some of the heterogeneity and explains the potential for synergism when two calcium antagonists are used concomitantly. In addition, these agents may also differ in their intracellular actions (on release of the calcium ion from the intracellular sarcoplasmic reticulum and the mitochondria as well as by binding with specific intracellular proteins such as calmodulin). As arteriolar resistance is diminished, total peripheral resistance is reduced and arterial pressure falls. However, one agent (nimodipine) has little effect on arterial pressure; its efficacy has been shown primarily for patients with cerebral bleeding.

Nine calcium antagonists are currently available in the US; a number of others are available elsewhere or their approval by the Food and Drugs Administration is imminent. Verapamil, in addition to its vasodilating property, has a cardiac inhibitory action, diminishing conduction and transmission. For this reason it was used initially for the treatment of supraventricular tachyarrhythmias (and was thought to be a beta-blocker). In contrast, nifedipine dilates arterioles; its cardiac effects are secondary to reflex stimulation (particularly with short-acting formulation). The longer-acting formulations of this latter compound are associated with less reflex cardiac stimulation and less pedal and dependent oedema. The other agents including diltiazem have fewer cardioinhibitory effects than verapamil, and may produce some reflex stimulation. All calcium antagonists reduce pressure without a consequent expansion of intravascular volume. This explains why they may be used as monotherapy for the treatment of hypertension. In part, this action is enhanced by the natriuretic effect of these agents as a result of their ability to inhibit renal tubular sodium reabsorption. As suggested above, some of these compounds have been associated with dependent pedal oedema related to the pressure reduction. However, it must be emphasized that this effect is related to potent precapillary arteriolar dilation with coexistent postcapillary reflex venoconstriction and increased hydrostatic pressure, favouring transcapillary migration of fluid into extravascular tissue. Thus, active renal fluid retention is a highly unlikely explanation for the oedema formation, and the natriuretic effect of these agents has been well documented.

All calcium antagonists have great similarity in their physiological antihypertensive action of decreased total peripheral resistance, except for nimodipine. The reduced vascular resistance seems to be distributed throughout the organ vasculatures, with the target organs of hypertension, heart, brain and kidney, sharing in this effect. These reduced organ vascular resistances may be associated with greater or lesser effects on organ flow, depending upon the agent employed. All agents appear to increase coronary blood flow, but diltiazem, amlodipine, felodipine and others also increase renal blood flow (probably through afferent and efferent glomerular dilation) without increasing glomerular filtration rate. Hence, they reduce renal filtration fraction, haemodynamic and glomerular actions that are not unlike those of ACE inhibitors or angiotensin II (type 1) receptor antagonists, although they are not operative through inhibition of the renin–angiotensin system. Indeed, renal micropuncture studies in various forms of experimental hypertension have demonstrated efferent glomerular arteriolar dilation and reduced glomerular hydrostatic. Most calcium antagonists reduce cardiac mass.

The calcium antagonists have been reported to be more efficacious in volume-dependent hypertensive patients with lower plasma renin activity and have been recommended for older or black patients with hypertension. Since there are no associated metabolic side-effects (e.g. hypokalaemia, carbohydrate intolerance, hyperlipidaemia, hyperuricaemia) with these compounds, they may be useful in those patients who have had these biochemical alterations with other antihypertensive agents. Calcium antagonists have not been associated with sexual dysfunction.

The Syst-Eur Study in Europe compared one calcium antagonist of the dihydropyridine group (nitrendipine, a compound unavailable in the US) with placebo treatment in elderly patients with isolated systolic hypertension. In that study, nitrendipine provided significant protection against stroke, although >25% of the patients received a concomitant diuretic and many others received a concomitant ACE inhibitor. Side-effects related to the calcium antagonists are constipation, flushing and headaches; in addition, gingival hyperplasia has been noted with most of these agents.

There has been controversy over the use of calcium antagonists following a report of a possibly greater likelihood of myocardial infarction in patients with hypertension treated with the short-acting formulations. The issue initially arose from a retrospective case study involving over 300 patients receiving these drugs, who were compared with over 2000 patients not receiving these agents. In part, the study reflects the drawbacks of retrospective case studies compared with the benefits of prospective, randomly assigned, double-blind trials. The study reported that the case study group of patients had a greater prevalence of complications from hypertensive and atherosclerotic vascular events prior to the initiation of antihypertensive therapy. But perhaps more important was the fact that only short-acting formulations of calcium antagonist were used. In short, the conclusions have not been confirmed in more recent studies which demonstrated improved end-points. Furthermore, the national and international guidelines have recommended use of calcium antagonists for patients with pre-existing cardiac involvement.

Morbidity and mortality

Until publication of JNC-V, VI and VII, the concept that specific antihypertensive agents significantly reduce total and cardiovascular morbidity and mortality had not been emphasized adequately. Much had been said in the earlier JNC reports about the efficacy of antihypertensive drug therapy and of their potential to reduce deaths and disability related to hypertension. Thus, a specific statement was made in JNC-V that the diuretics and beta-blockers 'are preferred because a reduction in morbidity and mortality has been demonstrated, and the other classes of antihypertensive agents have not yet been tested nor shown to reduce morbidity and mortality'. Unfortunately this statement led many to infer erroneously that only the diuretics and beta-blockers should be recommended for initial therapy of hypertension. On the contrary, it was made to highlight the wealth of clinical and epidemiological data that demonstrated only the diuretics and beta-adrenergic receptor blockers had been shown to reduce significantly the incidence of fatal and non-fatal strokes, myocardial infarction, congestive heart failure, accelerated and malignant hypertension, as well as progression of hypertensive disease to stages of greater severity. This statement was supported further by data from the European Working Party Study first report, and from other studies of elderly patients with diastolic hypertension, showing that treatment with methyldopa and diuretics was associated with fewer deaths from stroke and coronary heart disease. These findings were reinforced by other important reports demonstrating that diuretics and beta-blockers were also effective in reducing morbidity and mortality in elderly patients with isolated systolic hypertension.

Further reading

Joint National Committee on the Detection, Evaluation, and Treatment of Blood Pressure: The 1992 report of the Joint National Committee on the detection, evaluation, and treatment of blood pressure (JNC-V). *Arch. Intern. Med.* 1993;**153**: 154–183.

Joint National Committee on the Detection, Evaluation, and Treatment of High Blood Pressure: The sixth report of the Joint National Committee on prevention, detection, evaluation, and treatment of high blood pressure. *Arch. Intern. Med.* 1997;**157**:2413–2446. *These two references provide the basis for current national guidelines for the treatment of hypertension.*

Gurwitz JH, Bohn RL, Glynn RJ, Monane M, Mogun H, Avorn J: Antihypertensive drug therapy and the initiation of treatment for diabetes mellitus. *Ann. Intern. Med.* 1992;**118**:273–278.

Siscovick DS, Raghunathan TE, Psaty BM, *et al.*: Diuretic therapy for hypertension and the risk of primary cardiac arrest. *N. Engl. J. Med.* 1994;**330**:1852–1857. *Two excellent meta-analytic studies demonstrating the safety of low-dose thiazides with respect to sudden death and diabetes mellitus.*

Frohlich ED, Wilson IM, Schnaper HW, Freis ED: Hemodynamic alterations in hypertensive patients due to chlorothiazide. *N. Engl. J. Med.* 1960;**262**:1261–1263.

Freis ED, Wanko AM, Schnaper HW, Frohlic ED: Mechanism of the altered blood pressure responsiveness produced by chlorothiazide, *J. Clin. Invest.* 1960;**39**:1277–1281.

Frohlich, ED: Diuretics in hypertension. *J. Hypertens.* 1987;**5**(Suppl 3):S43-S49.

Frohlich ED: Inhibition of adrenergic function in the

treatment of hypertension. *Arch. Intern. Med.* 1974;**133**:1033–1048.

Frohlich ED: Methyldopa: mechanisms and treatment: 25 years later. *Arch. Intern. Med.* 1980;**140**:954–959.

Frohlich ED: Beta-adrenergic blockade in the circulatory regulation of hyperkinetic states. *Am. J. Cardiol.* 1971;**27**:195–199.

Frohlich ED: Beta-adrenergic receptor blockade in the treatment of essential hypertension. In: *The Heart in Hypertension.* BE Strauer (ed). Springer-Verlag, Berlin, 1981, pp. 425–435.

Aristizabal D, Frohlich ED: Calcium antagonists. In: *Cardiovascular Pharmacology and Therapeutics.* BN Singh, V Dzau, PM Vanhoutte, RL Woosley (eds). Churchill Livingstone, New York, 1993, pp. 185–202.

Frohlich ED: Angiotensin converting enzyme inhibitors: present and future. *Hypertension* 1989;**13**:125–130.

Frohlich ED, Iwata R, Sasaki O: Clinical and physiological significance of local tissue renin–angiotensin systems. *Am. J. Med.* 1989;**887**:19S–23S. *These eight references provide comprehensive reviews of various classes of antihypertensive therapies with lengthy bibliographies.*

Frohlich ED: Hypertension. In: *Conn's Current Therapy.* RE Rakel (ed). WB Saunders, Philadelphia, 2007, pp. 403–417.

Frohlich ED: Hypertension: essential. In: *Current Therapy in Cardiovascular Disease,* 4th edn. JW Hurst (ed). Mosby Year Book, Philadelphia, 1994, pp. 291–299. *These two references provide a concept of current antihypertensive drug therapy advocated by the author.*

Frohlich ED: The United States Joint National Committee's Recommendations: Its Fifth Report (1992). In: *Textbook of Hypertension.* JD Swales (ed). Blackwell Scientific Publications, Oxford, 1994, pp. 1203–1210. *A review of the various national programmes advocating initial therapy of hypertension.*

Laragh JH, Brenner BM (eds). *Hypertension: Pathophysiology, Diagnosis, and Management.* New York, Raven Press, 1995.

Kaplan NM: *Clinical Hypertension,* 7th edn. Baltimore, Williams and Wilkins, 1998. *These two references are the current and comprehensive textbooks on hypertension.*

Collins R. Peto R, MacMahon S, *et al.*: Blood pressure, stroke and coronary heart disease. II: Short-term reductions in blood pressure: overview of randomized drug trials in their epidemiological context. *Lancet* 1990;**335**:827–838.

Thijs L, Fagard R, Lijnen P, Staessen J, VanHoot R, Amery A: A meta-analysis of outcome trials in elderly hypertensives. *J. Hypertens.* 1992;**10**:1103–1109. *These two references provide the current meta-analyses of the early and most recent multicentre trials of antihypertensive therapy.*

SHEP Cooperative Research Group: Prevention of stroke by antihypertensive drug treatment in older persons with isolated systolic hypertension. *JAMA* 1991;**265**:3255–3264.

MRC Working Party: Medical Research Council trial of treatment of hypertension in older adults: principal results. *BMJ* 1992;**304**:405–412.

Dahlof B, Lindholm LH, Hansson L, Schersten B, Ekhom T, Wester PO: Morbidity and mortality in the Swedish Trial in Old Patients with Hypertension (STOP-Hypertension). *Lancet* 1991;**338**:1281–1285. *The last five references provide the supporting data for the feasibility and rationale for the treatment of isolated systolic hypertension in the elderly.*

Chapter 4

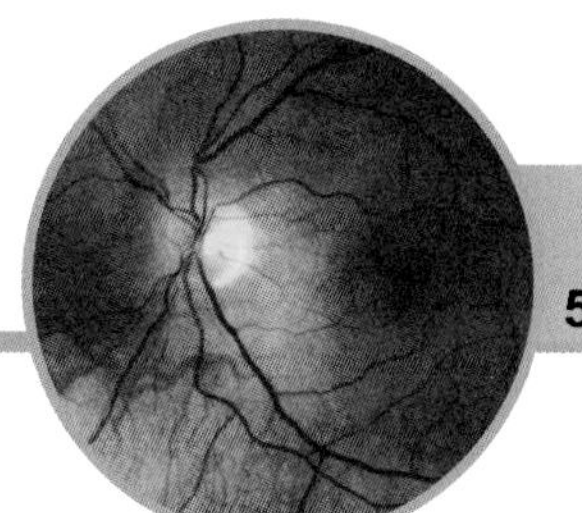

Uncomplicated essential hypertension

Introduction

Treatment of patients with essential hypertension has been tremendously successful since publication of the landmark Veterans Administrative Cooperative Study reports. With this impetus, guidelines for the detection, evaluation and treatment of hypertension were issued initially in 1970 by the National High Blood Pressure Education Program (NHBPEP) and were subsequently published by the first Joint National Committee Report (JNC-I) in 1972. The seventh of these guidelines was published in 2003; similar reports have been released by many other national and international consensus committees on the basis of advice from their respective expert organizations. Although these recommendations have been quite clear, they are also highly flexible and deal with uncomplicated essential hypertension as well as specific complications, target organ involvement, comorbid diseases, and other cardiovascular risk factors. Moreover, they are also applicable for patients with other (secondary) forms of systemic hypertension.

Following publication of JNC-I, the NHBPEP learned that only one-half of all people with hypertension were aware that their blood pressure was elevated. Of those who were aware that they had hypertension, one-half had received antihypertensive therapy and, of these, one-half had their blood pressure controlled. Thus, only 12.5% of the population with hypertension had optimal pressure control. Over the ensuing years there was progress in awareness, treatment and control of blood pressure. However, the most recent JNC-VII indicated real concern as the numbers of hypertensive patients detected, treated and controlled in 2003 had not improved satisfactorily (*Table 4.1*). The story elsewhere around the world is no better. Thus, the implications are clear: not enough is being done to control this major cardiovascular disease and risk factor underlying coronary heart disease.

In addition to disseminating the periodic JNC reports, the NHBPEP has promulgated many working group reports concerning specific hypertension-related problems. Among these are reports dealing with systolic hypertension; the heart, kidney, stroke and diabetes mellitus; hypertension in blacks, the elderly and paediatric and pregnant patients;

Table 4.1 Trends in awareness, treatment and control of high blood pressure in adults aged 18–74 years

	National Health and Nutrition Examination Survey (%)			
	II (1976–1980)	*III (Phase 1) (1988–1991)*	*III (Phase 2) (1991–1994)*	*1999–2000*
Awareness	51	73	68	70
Treatment	31	55	54	59
Control	10	29	27	34

non-pharmacological treatment; primary prevention; adherence; hypertension in the work setting; and others. Each report has been an important resource document for all health care professionals, the community, and third-party reimbursement organizations (see Further reading).

Classification and management of hypertension

At present, normal blood pressure is considered to be <120/<80 mmHg, systolic and diastolic, respectively (*Table 4.2*). Despite the normal, 'prehypertensive', or hypertensive ranges, all people should be encouraged to pursue healthy lifestyle patterns (see below).

Those individuals whose systolic and diastolic pressures range from 120 to 139 mmHg or from 80 to 89 mmHg, respectively, are said to have prehypertension. This range of pressure was formerly termed 'high normal' pressures. The choice of the term prehypertension has been strongly encouraged by epidemiologists and some others to help individuals to pursue lifestyle modification measures in order to prevent established or sustained essential hypertension from becoming manifest. However, the use of this term may serve to label normal individuals inappropriately as having hypertension. This has already prompted third party reimbursers to increase the insurance rate of some normotensives and even to reject some potential individuals from serving as renal (or other organ) donors.

Treatment of stage I and II hypertension

Patients with stage I hypertension (systolic pressures ranging from 140 to 159 mmHg or diastolic pressures from 90 to 99 mmHg documented on at least three separate occasions) should have their elevated pressures brought under control (<140 mmHg and <90 mmHg, systolic and diastolic, respectively). This may be approached initially with lifestyle (i.e. non-pharmacological approaches) modifications. If the elevated diastolic or systolic pressures are not controlled within a reasonable time (e.g. perhaps after 3–6 months but certainly less if the pressure elevation is associated with evidence of target organ involvement or a strong family history of premature cardiovascular death and disability), drug treatment is clearly indicated. In these individuals, particularly if significant demographic factors and comorbid diseases are present, vigorous antihypertensive treatment should be actively pursued (*Table 4.3*).

In patients with stage II hypertension (systolic pressure ≥160 mmHg or diastolic pressure ≥100 mmHg), pharmacological therapy should probably be initiated at the outset (after satisfactory confirmation), together with specific and detailed advice to modify lifestyle practices. As indicated below, many reports have demonstrated not only that lifestyle modification measures may provide control of low-grade pressure elevations but also that in patients with

Table 4.2 Classification of blood pressure

Classification	*Systolic (mmHg)*	*Diastolic (mmHg)*	*Lifestyle modifications*	*Initial drug therapy without compelling indications*
Normal	<120 and	<80	Encourage	None
Prehypertension	120–139	or 80–89	Yes	None
Stage I hypertension	140–159	or 90–99	Yes	Thiazide-type diuretic and/or beta-blocker; may consider ACE inhibitor, angiotensin receptor blocker, renin inhibitor, calcium antagonists or combination
Stage II hypertension	≥160	or ≥100	Yes	Usually two-drug combination or any of the above with more frequent follow-up and additional agents to the initial selection until blood pressure is controlled

higher pressure elevations lifestyle changes will reduce the number of drugs (or their doses) required. By the same token, many other studies have demonstrated that most patients with hypertension who have discontinued therapy must subsequently resume pharmacological therapy.

Table 4.3 Indications for initiating pharmacological therapy in patients with prehypertension or stage I hypertension

- Positive family history of cardiovascular disease with premature death
- Failure of pressure to respond to lifestyle modifications
- Evidence of target organ involvement:
  - Heart
    a. Left ventricular hypertrophy
    b. Cardiac failure
    c. Cardiac dysrhythmias
    d. Electrocardiographic changes
    e. Angina pectoris
    f. Myocardial infarction
  - Kidney
    a. Renal functional impairment
    b. Persistent proteinuria
    c. Possibly polycystic renal disease
    d. Possibly occlusive renal arterial diseases (fibrosing, atherosclerotic)
  - Brain
    a. Hypertensive retinopathy
    b. Transient ischaemic attacks
    c. Stroke
- Related comorbid diseases or cardiovascular risk factors:
  - Carbohydrate intolerance/diabetes mellitus
  - Hyperlipidaemia
  - Exogenous obesity
  - Atherosclerosis
  - Tobacco addiction
- Significant demographic factors:
  - Male gender
  - Black race

Selection of initial therapy

Non-pharmacological (lifestyle modification) approaches

Since publication of JNC-III, non-pharmacological approaches have been recommended as a basis upon which further (pharmacological) therapy is prescribed (*Table 4.4*). Many studies have demonstrated clearly that with weight control (to ideal body weight levels; BMI, 18.5–24.9), sodium restriction (<100 mmol [mEq] daily), alcohol moderation (<1 oz ethanol or its equivalent daily), aerobic exercise (at least 20 minutes, 3 days a week), and adequate dietary intake of potassium, blood pressure might be fully controlled in patients with small pressure elevation. Smoking cessation promotes good overall cardiovascular health and effectiveness of prescribed antihypertensive therapy. Indeed, several studies have shown that the smoker does not have the same protection from death, stroke or coronary heart disease as the non-smoker, nor does the smoker who is receiving a diuretic and whose blood pressure level is similarly controlled.

Pharmacological therapy

Any of the currently recommended classes of drugs may be chosen for initial antihypertensive therapy.

Table 4.4 Lifestyle modifications for hypertension

For prevention and management

- Lose weight if overweight or obese
- Reduce sodium intake
- Limit alcohol intake
- Increase aerobic physical activity.
- Maintain adequate potassium intake

For overall and cardiovascular health

- Stop smoking (see text)
- Reduce dietary saturated fat and cholesterol
- Maintain adequate intake of calcium and magnesium

Obesity

The term 'factors of risk' was first introduced by the Framingham Heart Study almost five decades ago to identify demographically specific clinical characteristics that confer increased risk of cardiovascular morbidity and mortality. Initially encompassing only four risk factors, the factors of risk comprise hypertension, hyperlipidaemia, left ventricular hypertrophy, diabetes mellitus, smoking, exogenous obesity, several non-modifiable factors including age, black race and male gender, some less established factors that include hyperuricaemia and hyperfibrinogenaemia, and certain currently investigated 'biomarkers' that are end-points of cardiovascular diseases. Obesity is associated with increased intravascular (plasma) volume, which in turn is associated with increased venous return to the heart and cardiac output and increased blood flow and cardiac output to kidneys and other organs in both normal and hypertensive subjects. These haemodynamic derangements are associated with structural changes that include deposition of fat around the major organs such as the heart and kidney. Thus, and most importantly, obesity results in an increased intra-vascular volume and pressure overload on the heart, which increase the risk of hypertension.

Salt

Salt has played an important role in the social, economic and other aspects of human existence for millennia. However, over the past 100 years, medical practitioners have become increasingly interested in the role of salt excess in disease. More specifically, the adverse effect of salt or sodium excess has captured broad attention because of its direct role in cardiovascular and renal diseases and their outcomes. Stimulated by repeated epidemiological studies that have shown a strongly positive association between the magnitude of salt consumption and the prevalence of hypertensive diseases, many fundamental and clinical studies have focused on the potential mechanisms that might explain this association. However, only about one-third of patients with essential hypertension demonstrate increased 'salt sensitivity'. Our imagination has been provoked by the possibility that salt excess might not only increase arterial pressure, but might even enhance the pathophysiological changes of hypertensive disease in addition to, and independent of, its effect on arterial pressure. Thus, we have demonstrated experimentally in our laboratory that salt excess produces diastolic dysfunction associated with deposition of collagen in the extracellular matrix and perivascularly in the ventricle; diminished aortic distensibility; and, in renal failure associated with diminished renal blood flow, afferent and efferent glomerular arteriolar constriction with increased glomerular hydrostatic pressure and severe arteriolar and glomerular injury. Most of these findings have been confirmed in humans.

Diuretics

The thiazide diuretics have been recommended for initial pharmacological monotherapy of hypertension ever since promulgation of the very first guidelines were published. The rationale for their use was not based solely on clinical empiricism, but on strong clinical evidence and, just as important, on sound physiological rationale. Were anti-hypertensive treatment to be initiated with either of the two oldest antihypertensive drug classes (i.e. adrenergic inhibitors, smooth muscle relaxants), following an initial reduction in the blood pressure, the pressure would most likely return to on or around pretreatment values. The mechanism for this is not 'drug tolerance' to these agents; intravascular (i.e. plasma) volume expands as a consequence of pressure reduction ('pseudotolerance'). Diuretic monotherapy has its own intrinsic ability to reduce (if not control) arterial pressure in 15–50% of patients with essential hypertension (depending upon the initial pressures of the population group studied).

The various options for diuretic agents are:

- Thiazides.
- Thiazide congeners.
- Potassium-retaining agents.
- Loop-acting agents.

Generally, the thiazide agents (e.g. chlorothiazide, hydrochlorothiazide) are recommended, and the thiazide congeners (e.g. chlorthalidone) have also been used for several decades and in several multicentre studies. *Table 4.5* presents patients who might be selected for initial thiazide monotherapy.

The more common biochemical effects of the drugs are listed in *Table 4.6*; but, as discussed in Chapter 4, they are less likely to occur with a low initial dose (e.g. hydrochlorothiazide 12.5–25 mg daily), which can be increased to 25 or even 50 mg. These considerations and other details are discussed in Chapter 5, including the risk of hypoglycaemia and sudden cardiac death. With the addition or initial selection of agents from other antihypertensive drug classes, effective pressure

Table 4.5 Selection of patients for initial treatment with thiazides

- Elderly
- Black race
- Obese
- Female
- Volume dependent
- Low plasma renin activity
- Steroid dependent
- Renal disease
- Isolated systolic hypertension

Table 4.6 Biochemical effects of thiazides

- Hypokalaemia
- Hyponatraemia
- Carbohydrate intolerance
- Impaired renal function
- Hyperuricaemia
- Hyperlipidaemia
- Hypocalcaemia
- Hypomagnesaemia

Table 4.7 Beta-blockers for use in uncomplicated essential hypertension

Non-selective	*Cardioselective*	*Intrinsic sympathomimetic activity*
	Atenolol	Acebutalol
	Metoprolol	Pindolol
Betaxolol	Timolol	Renbutol
Bisoprolol		
Celiprolol		
Esmolol (i.v. only)		
Nadolol		
Propranolol		
Alpha-1 and beta-adrenergic receptor inhibitors		
Labetalol		
Carvedilol		

control may be expected in upwards of 85% of patients with lower doses of diuretics. This therapeutic manoeuvre serves to reduce the development of side-effects from other agents or even higher doses of the added agent. It is noteworthy, however, that the addition of a diuretic to a calcium antagonist may not be very effective in reducing pressure further. Perhaps this explains why these two classes of drugs are not available as combination therapy.

Beta-adrenergic receptor inhibitors

This class of antihypertensive agents has been recommended for initial therapy because abundant experience has indicated that beta-blockers can be prescribed without the likelihood of intravascular volume expansion, loss of arterial pressure control, and with predictable effectiveness in a significant population (but not all) of hypertensive patients. Moreover, their antihypertensive effectiveness may be increased further with the addition of a diuretic. The various options of beta-blockers (*Table 4.7*) and the patients most likely to be selected for therapy (*Table 4.8*) are presented.

In recent years some authorities have expressed their opinion that these beta-blockers do not merit consideration for prescription as initial therapy. However, we do not accept this concept. The arguments advanced by the former thought-leaders are based upon experiences derived from groups of patients or by meta-analysis. In our experience there are individual patients who are more likely to respond

Table 4.8 Selection of patients for initial treatment with beta-blockers

- White race
- Male
- Hyperdynamic circulation
- Angina pectoris
- Prior myocardial infarction
- Mitral valve prolapse (idiopathic)
- Cardiac dysrhythmias (responsive to beta-blockers)
- Migraine headaches

to beta-blockers alone (see **4.8**). In particular, they include patients with a hyperdynamic circulation; younger patients with a lesser degree of blood pressure elevation; and patients with certain cardiac dysrhythmias, mitral valvular prolapse (idiopathic), angina pectoris or prior myocardial infarction.

The clinical pharmacological characteristics of this class of agents are discussed in greater detail in Chapter 5; a summary of the mechanisms of action (*Table 4.9*) and side-effects (*Table 4.10*) are presented in Tables 4.9 and 4.10.

Alpha-1-adrenergic and alpha–beta adrenergic receptor inhibitors

Although suggested in earlier JNC reports, the alpha-1-adrenergic and the alpha–beta adrenergic receptor inhibitors have been recommended for initial monotherapy. These agents are effective in controlling arterial pressure but may be associated with expanded intravascular (plasma) volume (i.e. pseudotolerance). Because of this, peripheral oedema may occur and could be associated with symptoms suggesting cardiac failure. For this reason, doxazosin was removed from the ALLHAT study, with the statement that cardiac failure occurred with increased frequency compared with the other agents in that study (i.e. chlorthalidone, lisinopril and amlodipine). Nevertheless, alpha-1-adrenergic receptor inhibitors have continued to be used by patients with prostatic hyperplasia; concerns regarding further blood pressure reduction or postural hypotension have been raised, and falls with possible bone fractures have occurred. An alpha-1-adrenergic inhibitor has been made available (relatively recently) for normotensive patients with benign prostatic hyperplasia, which does not seem to be as potent in reducing arterial pressure.

Table 4.9 Mechanism of action of beta-adrenergic receptor inhibitors

- Reduced heart rate and cardiac output
- Varying effects on organ blood flows:
  - Depending on beta-receptor density
- Reduced plasma renin activity
- No expansion of plama volume
- Reduced left ventricular mass
- Protection against second myocardial infarction

Table 4.10 Side-effects of beta-blocker therapy

- Reduced pulmonary airway flow
  - Asthma
  - Obstructive lung disease
- Bradycardia and potential increase in first-degree heart block
- Peripheral arterial insufficiency
- Depression
- Metabolic
  - Increased triglycerides
  - Decreased high-density lipoprotein

Alpha–beta adrenergic receptor inhibitors may be used with the expectation of greater reductions of blood pressure. Their effectiveness is also increased with the addition of diuretic. A newer alpha–beta adrenergic receptor blocker (corvedilol) has greater beta-receptor blocking activity than alpha, and has been shown in a large multicentre study (COPERNICUS) to be of additional value in the treatment of cardiac failure (particularly in non-hypertensive patients). Moreover, this agent has been suggested to have putative anti-inflammatory actions.

Calcium antagonists

Controlled multicentre trials (Syst-Eur, STONE) have shown that certain calcium antagonists have been of value in elderly patients with isolated systolic hypertension, and provide protection from fatal and non-fatal strokes. Specifically, nitrendipine (unavailable in the US) reduced mortality from strokes in the well-controlled Syst-Eur study (**4.1**); long-acting nifedipine did likewise in the STONE trial, although the design of this study has been criticized (by some). Additionally, amlodipine provides equal (or slightly better) control of arterial pressure than an angiotensin II (type 1) receptor blocker with similar efficacy. Thus, all dihydropyridine calcium antagonists (nitrendipine is one) have been considered for initial treatment and protection from stroke.

As discussed in Chapter 3, the calcium antagonists are a very heterogeneous class of drugs with respect to chemical structure and pharmacological and physiological actions (*Table 4.11*). To date, five calcium channel receptors have been cloned. Since the drugs act not only at these five extracellular channel receptor sites, but also intracellularly on calcium ion release from intracellular stores from the sarcoplasmic reticulum, the mitochondria, or from intracellular proteins (**4.2**), the International Pharmacological Union prefers to use the nomenclature of calcium antagonists over the common term, calcium channel blockers.

The clinician should be aware that nifedipine also binds to alpha-adrenergic receptor sites; that nimodipine does not reduce arterial pressure at all but has preference for cerebral vasodilation; and that some calcium antagonists may have greater preference for renal dilatation (e.g. diltiazem, verapamil and some dihydropyridines produce afferent as well as efferent glomerular arteriolar dilation, thereby

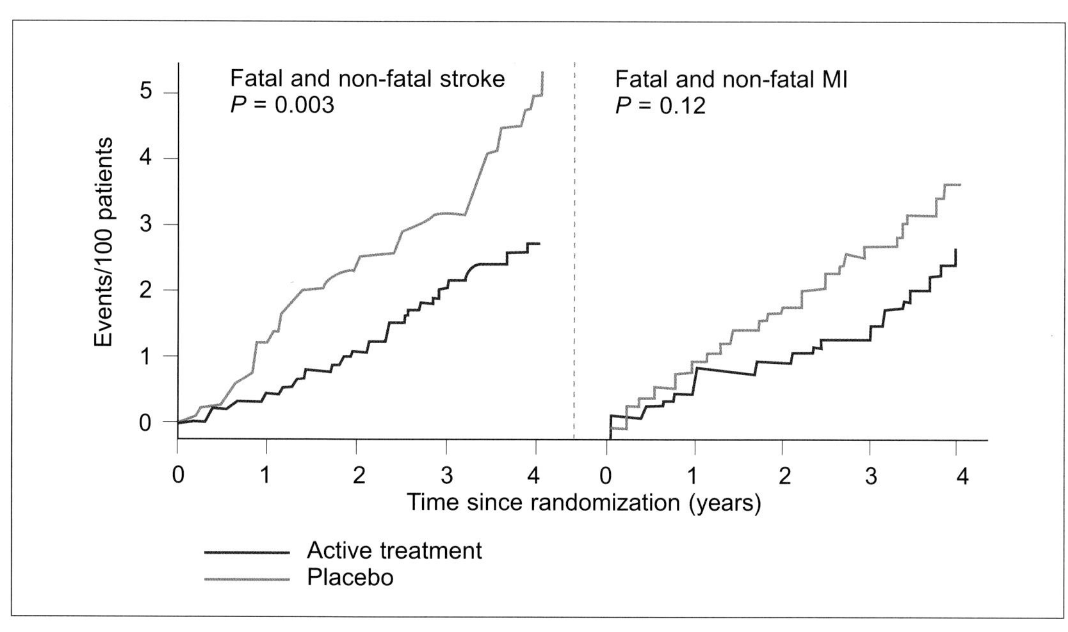

4.1 Cumulative rates of fatal and non-fatal strokes and myocardial infarction by treatment group. These findings were reported with nitrendipine in the Sys-Eur study.

Table 4.11 Calcium antagonists used in the treatment of uncomplicated essential hypertension

• Amlodipine	• Gallopamil	• Nimodipine
• Clentiazem	• Isradipine	• Nisoldipine
• Diltiazem	• Nicardipine	• Nitrendipine
• Felodipine	• Nifedipine	• Verapamil

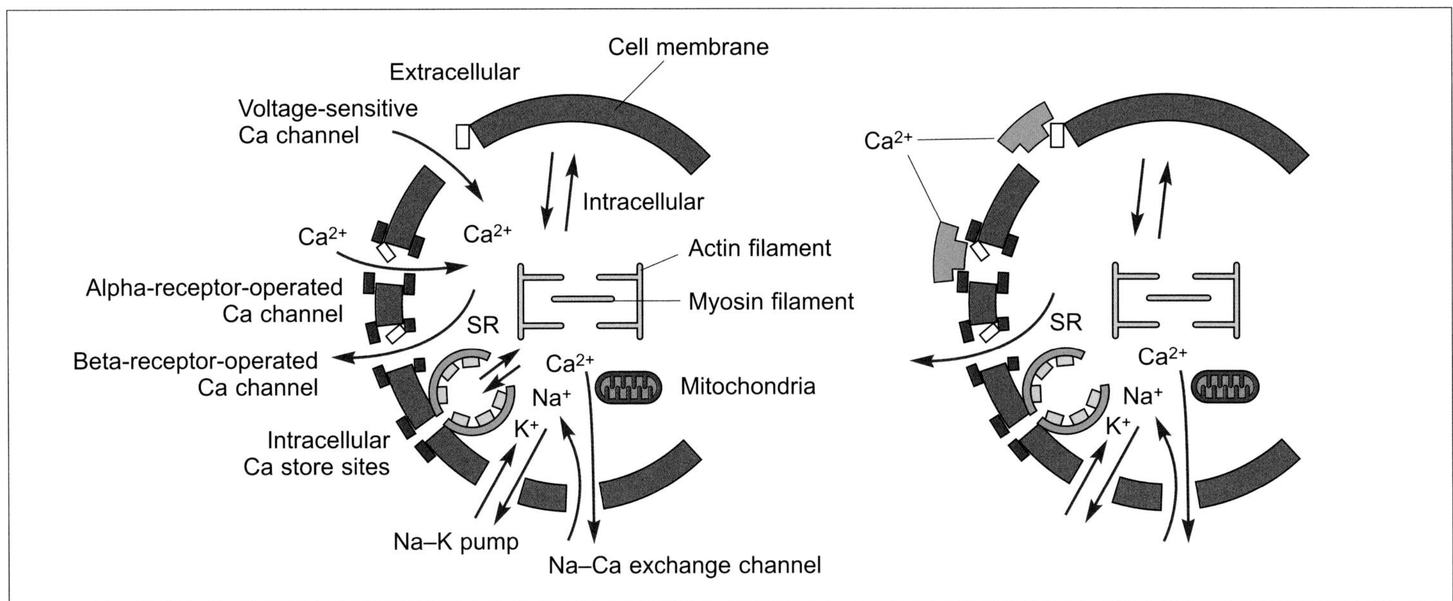

4.2 Sites of action of calcium antagonists on vascular smooth muscle. (From Aoki and Salto.)

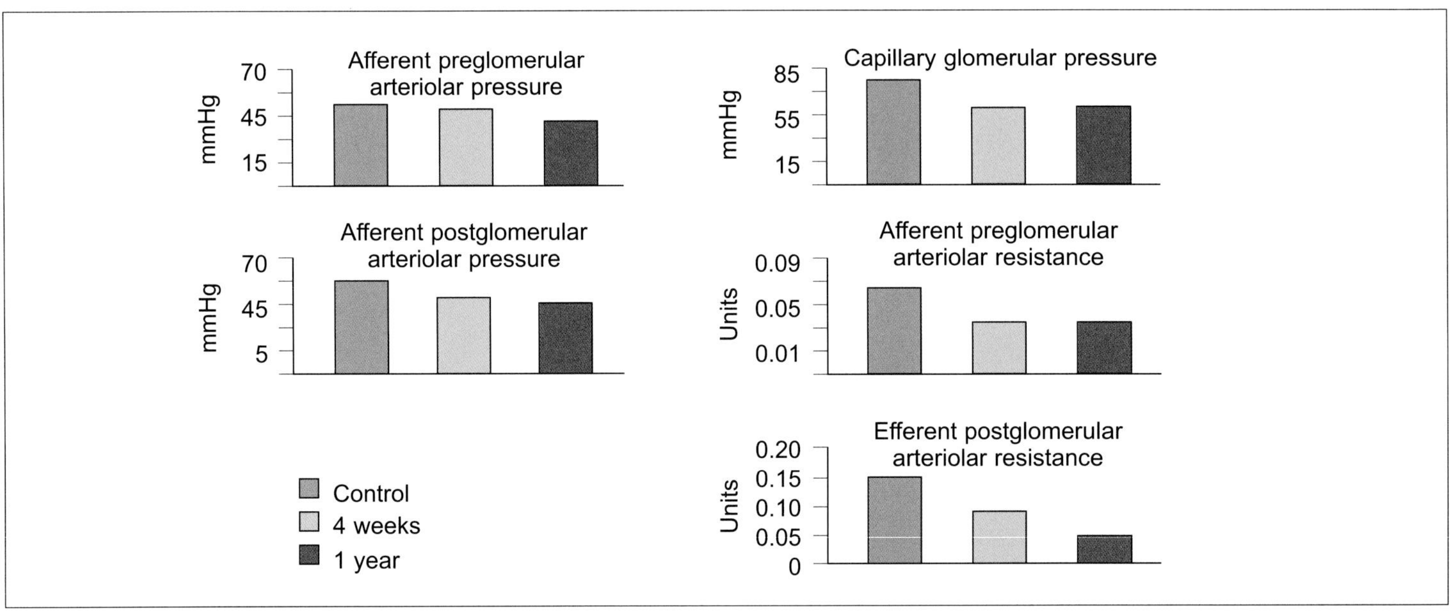

4.3 Effects of prolonged diltiazem (300 mg/day). **A**: intrarenal dynamics; **B**: haemodynamics.

reducing glomerular hydrostatic pressure) (**4.3**). Calcium antagonist antihypertensive agents are discussed more fully in Chapter 3. A summary of the general mechanisms of action and a guide for selection of patients for initial treatment are provided in *Tables 4.12* and *4.13*, respectively.

Angiotensin-converting enzyme inhibitors

The angiotensin-converting enzyme (ACE) inhibitors are also excellent for initial monotherapy. Intravascular (i.e. plasma) volume expansion does not occur with these agents, even though the addition of a diuretic may further enhance their antihypertensive effectiveness. A number of multicentre trials have demonstrated conclusively that they are highly effective for the treatment of hypertensive patients with renal functional impairment or end-stage renal disease (ESRD). When initially reported for patients with diabetes mellitus (with or without hypertension), progression of renal functional impairment and ESRD was retarded significantly

Table 4.12 Mechanism of action of calcium antagonists

- Reduced intramyocytic Ca^{2+}
- Reduced vascular resistance
- Potentially reduced cardiac chronotropic and inotropic effects
- (Usually) little reflex cardiac stimulation
- Variable organ flow responses
- No expansion of plasma volume
- Reduced left ventricular mass

Table 4.13 Selection of patients for initial treatment with calcium antagonists

- Elderly
- Black race
- Angina pectoris
- Prior myocardial infarction
- Atherosclerosis regression
- Bilateral renal arterial disease
- Metabolic alterations precluding other therapy
- Side-effects with other therapy
- Left ventricular hypertrophy
- Renal parenchymal disease
- ?Volume dependent with hypertension

and the necessity for haemodialysis was reduced significantly. Moreover, the ACE inhibitors have been shown to reduce morbidity and mortality in patients with myocardial infarction. In these studies, the drugs were also shown to prevent (or at least reduce the development) of congestive heart failure and death following myocardial infarction. Although these studies were conducted primarily in normotensive patients, some hypertensive and previously hypertensive patients were included. Therefore, it is reasonable to expect similar findings in patients with hypertension. The ACE inhibitors are recommended for initial use at low doses, and may subsequently be increased to full dosage. Of course, a second pharmacological agent could be added to the initially selected agent for the overall treatment programme. (Already suggested a diuretic but also a calcium antagonist.)

Angiotensin II (type 1) receptor blockers (ARBs) and the renin inhibitors

Angiotensin II (type 1) receptor antagonists are recommended for initial treatment of hypertension. Unlike the ACE inhibitors, these agents do not produce cough since they do not work through ACE inhibition and the increase of kinin (which may be the mechanism producing the ACE inhibition cough). A number of multicentre trials have demonstrated the efficacy of the ARBs in cardiac failure, stroke, and in renal involvement (related to diabetes mellitus and hypertension).

Renin inhibitors

At the time of writing, only one pharmacological agent (aliskiren; US tradename Tekturna) directly inhibits the rate-limiting biochemical step by impairing the ability of renin to promote the conversion of angiotensinogen to angiotensin I. As a consequence, the cascading effects of the renin–angiotensin–aldosterone system are markedly inhibited. Clinical experience with this new compound is only just beginning, but the following information seems to be well established. The drug reduces arterial pressure in a dose-dependent fashion, suppresses plasma renin activity in combination with a diuretic and is approved for once-daily oral administration. In addition, the agent is clinically safe and effective when used alone as well as with other anti-hypertensive agents (e.g. a diuretic, calcium antagonist, ACE inhibitor, an ARB). To date, there have been no major adverse effects and, because it has no action on the angiotensin-converting enzyme, treatment is not associated with cough but angioneurotic odema remains a concern and hyperkalaemia is still possible if this agent is used with an ACE inhibitor or an ARB. Thus, this agent will be useful in the treatment of patients with essential hypertension and holds great promise for patients with renal functional impairment because of its antiproteinuric effects experimentally.

Combination therapy

A number of low-dose drug combinations are especially

appropriate therapies for certain 'compelling indications' in the initial treatment of patients with hypertension (see subsequent chapters). These include thiazide diuretic with potassium-sparing agent; diuretic with beta-blocker, ACE inhibitor, or angiotensin II (type 1 receptor antagonist); and calcium antagonist with ACE inhibitor; methyldopa or clonidine with diuretic; prazosin with diuretic; and others.

Reducing morbidity and mortality

The JNC committees (since JNC-V) were cognizant that the efficacy of antihypertensive therapy to reduce total and cardiovascular morbidity and mortality had not been sufficiently emphasized in prior decision-making processes for selecting initial options for monotherapy of hypertension. Furthermore, this concept is of particular relevance when disease outcome events resulting from therapeutic intervention are becoming important in formulating treatment algorithms. This is very important even though much had been highlighted earlier about the efficacy of antihypertensive therapy and its potential to reduce deaths and disability related to hypertension and its complications. For this reason, an algorithm for initial therapy of hypertension was included in JNC-V, reiterated in JNC-VI (**4.4**).

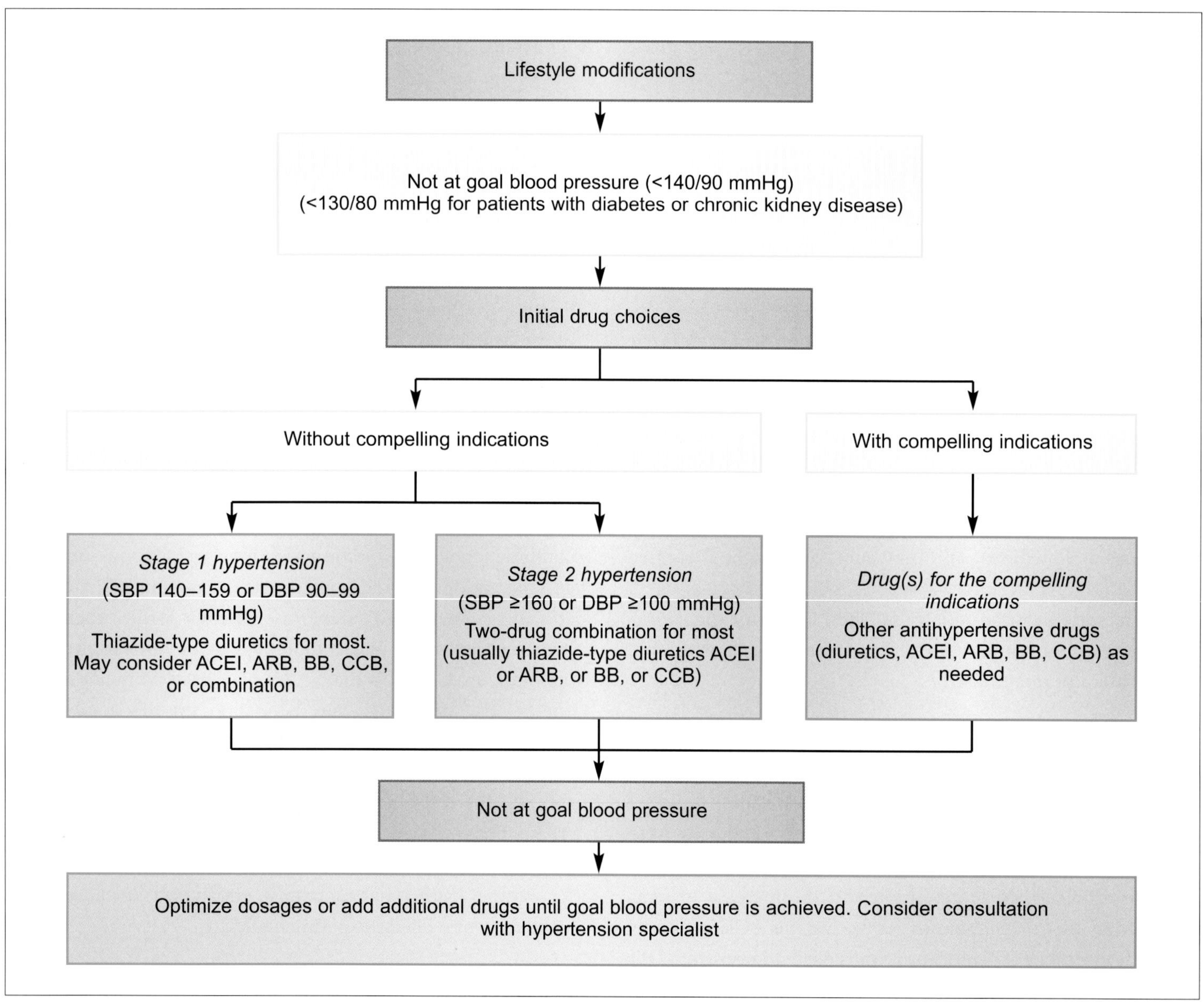

4.4 Algorithm for the initial therapy of hypertension. (DBP, diastolic blood pressure; SBP, systolic blood pressure; ACEI, angiotensin-converting enzyme inhibitor; ARB, angiotensin receptor blocker; BB, beta-blocker; CCB, calcium channel blocker [calcium antagonists].) (Adapted from *JAMA* 2003; **289**:2560–2572.)

The rationale for stating that diuretics were the preferred agents (as also discussed in Chapter 3) was made to emphasize the tremendous body of epidemiological data that had accumulated with these agents over more than four decades, which demonstrated a significant reduction in fatal and non-fatal strokes, myocardial infarction, congestive heart failure, development of accelerated and malignant hypertension, and progression in severity of hypertensive disease. Moreover, these findings were reinforced by subsequent reports of their efficacy in large trials, demonstrating reduction in morbidity and mortality in elderly patients with isolated systolic hypertension.

However, the other seven classes of agents (beta-blockers, ACE inhibitors, angiotensin receptor blockers, renin inhibitors, calcium antagonists, alpha- and alpha–beta blockers) are as effective in controlling elevated arterial pressure in hypertension. Thus, if the physician believes that any of these other classes of agents would be more beneficial for a specific patient or if other clinical and therapeutic considerations exist, selection from these other classes is clearly appropriate. This rationale may include a simpler treatment protocol, consideration of prior responses to antihypertensive therapy, the patient's overall medical status including comorbid diseases and cardiovascular risk factors, side-effects of other agents, and simplification in patient management (including the need for other drugs, laboratory test, and missed time from work for follow-up).

In providing a rationale for selecting initial monotherapy for hypertension, the successive JNC reports have included a detailed listing and discussion of each of the classes and combinations of antihypertensive agents, their usual daily dosages (*Tables 4.14–4.20*), mechanisms of action and comparative efficacy. (See chapters on clinical pharmacology for discussion of side-effects). It is well known that diuretics have certain metabolic effects (*Table 4.6*). Each class of agents has been identified in either earlier and more

Table 4.14 Joint National Committee-VII guidelines for the prescribing of diuretics

Class	*Generic (trade) name*	*Daily dose (mg)*
Thiazides	Bendroflumethiazide (Methahydrin)	2.5–5.0
	Benzthiazide (Aquatagiexna)	125–500
	Chlorothiazide (Diuril)	125–500
	Chlorthalidone	12.5–25
	Hydrochlorothiazide (Microzide, HydroDiuril)	12.5–50.0
	Hydroflumethiazide (Saluron)	2.5–10.0
	Indapamide (Lozol)	1.25–2.5
	Metolazone (Mykrox)	0.5–1.0
	Metolazone (Zaroxolyn)	1.0–4.0
	Microzide	2.5–5.0
	Naturetin	12.5–50.0
	Polythiazide (Renese)	2.0–4.0
Loop agents	Bumetanide (Bumex)	0.5–2.0
	Ethacrynic acid (Edecrin)	25–100
	Furosemide (Lasix)	20–80
	Tosemide (Demadex)	2.5–10.0
Potassium-sparing agents	Amiloride (Midamor)	5.0–10.0
	Triamterene (Dyrenium)	50–100
Aldosterone receptor blockers	Eplerenone (Inspra)	50–100
	Spironolactone (Aldactone)	25–50

Table 4.15 Joint National Committee-VII guidelines for the prescribing of beta-blockers in uncomplicated essential hypertension

Subclass	*Generic (trade) name*	*Daily dose (mg)*
Beta-adrenergic receptor blockers (without intrinsic sympathomimetic activity)	Atenolol (Tenormin)	25–100
	Betaxolol (Kerlone)	5–20
	Bisoprolol (Zebeta)	2.5–10.0
	Esmolol (Brevibloc)	i.v.
	Metoprolol (Lopressor)	50–100 qd or bid
	Metoprolol extended release (Toprol XL)	50–100
	Nadolol (Corgard)	40–120
	Propranolol (Inderal)	40–160 qd or bid
	Propranolol long-acting (Inderal LA)	60–180
	Timolol (Blocadren)	20–40 qd or bid
With intrinsic sympathomimetic activity	Acebutolol (Sectral)	200–800 qd or bid
	Pindolol	10–40 qd or bid
	Renbutolol (Levatol)	10–40
Combined alpha–beta-adrenergic receptor blockers	Carvedilol (Coreg)	12.5–40 bid
	Labetalol (Normodyne, Trandate)	200–800 bid

Table 4.16 Joint National Committee-VII guidelines for the prescribing of alpha-1-receptor blockers, centrally acting and other adrenergic inhibitors, and direct-acting smooth muscle vasodilators in uncomplicated essential hypertension

Class of agent	*Generic (trade) name*	*Daily dose (mg)*
Alpha-1 blockers	Doxazosin (Cardura)	1.0–10.0
	Prazosin (Minipress)	2.0–20.0 bid or tid
	Terazosin (Hydrin)	1.0–20.0 qd or bid
Alpha-1 pre- and postsynaptic receptor blockers	Phentolamine (Regitine)	5.0–10.0
	Phenoxybenzamine (Dibenzyline)	10–40
Central alpha-2 agonists and other centrally acting agents	Clonidine (Catapres)	0.1–0.8 bid
	Clonidine patch (Catapres-TTS)	0.1–0.3 weekly
	Methyldopa (Aldomet)	250–1000 bid
	Reserpine (generic)	0.1–0.25 qd
	Guanfacine (Tenex)	0.5–2.0 qd
Direct-acting vasodilators	Hydralazine (Apresoline)	25–100 bid or tid
	Minoxidil (Loniten)	2.5–80 qd or bid

Table 4.17 Joint National Committee-VII guidelines for the prescribing of calcium antagonists in uncomplicated essential hypertension

Class	*Generic (Trade) name*	*Daily dose (mg)*
Nondihydropyridines	Diltiazem extended release (Cardizem CD, Dilacor XR, Tiazac)	180–420
	Diltiazem extended release (Cardizem LA)	120–540
	Verapamil immediate release (Calan, Isoptin)	80–320 qd or bid
	Verapamil long-acting (Calan SR, Isoptin SR)	120–480 qd or bid
	Verapamil-Coer, (Covera HS, Verelan PM)	120–360
Dihydropyridines	Amlodipine (Norvasc)	2.5–10.0
	Felodipine (Plendil)	2.5–20
	Isradipine (Dynacirc (CR)	2.5–10.0 bid
	Nifedipine long-acting (Adalat CC, Procardia XL)	30–60
	Nisoldipine (Sular)	10–40

Table 4.18 Joint National Committee-VII guidelines for the prescribing of angiotensin-converting enzyme inhibitors and angiotensin II receptor antagonists in uncomplicated essential hypertension

Subgroup	*Generic (Trade) name*	*Daily dose (mg)*
Angiotensin-converting enzyme inhibitors	Benazepril (Lotensin)	10–40
	Captopril (Capoten)	25–100
	Enalapril (Vasotec)	5–40 qd or bid
	Fosinopril (Monopril)	10–40
	Lisinopril (Prinivil, Zentril)	10–40
	Moexipril (Univasc)	7.5–30.0
	Perindopril (Aceon)	4.0–8.0
	Quinapril (Accuptil)	10–80
	Ramipril (Altace)	2.5–20.0
	Trandolapril (Mavik)	1.0–4.0
Angiotensin II (type 1) receptor antagonists	Candesartan (Atacand)	8–32
	Eprosartan (Teveten)	400–800 qd or bid
	Irbesartan (Avapro)	150–300
	Losartan (Cozaar)	25–100 qd or bid
	Olmesartan (Benicar)	20–40
	Telmisartan (Micardis)	20–80
	Valsartan (Diovan)	80–320 qd or bid

Table 4.19 Joint National Committee-VII guidelines for the prescribing of fixed-dose combinations of diuretics with beta-blockers or other agents in uncomplicated essential hypertension

Class	*Combination*	*Trade name (US)*
Beta-adrenergic receptor blocker with diuretic	Atenolol–chlorthalidone (50/25, 100/25)	Tenoretic
	Bisoprolol–hydrochlorothiazide (2.5/6.25, 5/6.25, 10/6.25)	Ziac
	Metoprolol–hydrochlorothiazide (50/25, 100/25)	Lopressor HCT
	Nadolol–bendroflumethiazide (40/5, 80/5)	Corzide
	Propranolol LA–hydrochlorothiazide (40/25, 80/25)	Inderide LA
Diuretic and potassium-retaining agent	Amiloride–hydrochlorothiazide (5/50)	Moduretic
	Spironolactone–hydrochlorothiazide (25/25, 50/50)	Aldactiazide
	Triamterene–hydrochlorothiazide (37.5/25, 75/50)	Dyazide, Maxzide
Centrally acting agent and diuretic	Methyldopa–hydrochlorothiazide (250/15, 250/25, 500/30, 500/50)	Aldoril
	Reserpine-chlothalidone (0.125/25, 0.25/50)	Demi-Regroton, Regroton
	Reserpine–chlorothiazide (0.125/250, 0.25/500)	Diupres
	Reserpine–hydrochlorothiazide (0.125/25, 0.125/50)	Hydropres

Table 4.20 Joint National Committee-VII guidelines for the prescribing of fixed-dose combinations of angiotensin-converting enzyme inhibitors or angiotensin receptor blockers with other agents in uncomplicated essential hypertension

Class	*Combination*	*Trade name (US)*
Angiotensin-converting enzyme inhibitor and diuretic	Benazepril–hydrochlorothiazide (5/6.25, 10/12.5, 20/12.5, 20/25)	Lotensin HCT
	Captopril–hydrochlorothiazide (25/l5,25/25, 50/15, 50/25)	Capozide
	Enalapril–hydrochlorothiazide (5/12.5, 10/25)	Vaseretic
	Fosinopril–hydrochlorothiazide (10/12.5, 20/12.5)	Monopril HCT
	Lisinopril–hydrochlorothiazide (10/12.5, 202/12.5, 20/25)	Prinzide, Zestoretic
	Moexipril–hydrochlorothiazide (7.5/12.5, 15/25)	Uriretic
	Quinapril–hydrochlorothiazide (10/12.5, 20/12.5, 20/25)	Accuretic
Angiotensin-converting enzyme inhibitor and calcium antagonist	Amlodipine–benazepril hydrochloride (2.5/10, 5/10, 5/20, 10/20)	Lotrel
	Enalapril–felodipine (5/5)	Lexxel
	Trandolapril–verapamil (2/180, 1/240, 2/240, 4/240)	Tarka
Angiotensin II receptor antagonist and diuretic	Candesartan–hydrochlorothiazide (16/12.5, 32/12.5)	Atacand HCT
	Eprosartan–hydrochlorothiazide (600/12.5, 600/25)	Teveten HCT
	Ibersartan–hydrochlorothiazide (150/12.5, 600/25)	Avalide
	Losartan–hydrochlorothiazide (50/12.5, 100/25)	Hyzaar
	Olmesartan medoxomil–hydrochlorothiazide (20/12.5, 40/12.5, 40/25)	Benicar HCT
	Telmisartan–hydrochlorothiazide (40/12.5, 80/12.5)	Micardis HCT
	Valsartan–hydrochlorothiazide (80/12.5, 160/12.25, 160/25)	Diovan HCT

recent multicentre studies that have demonstrated reduced morbidity and mortality. However, in the earlier studies, the diuretics were prescribed in much higher doses than those employed in more recent trials (e.g. hydrochlorothiazide 50 mg twice daily vs. 12.5–25 mg daily, with the later full dose as 50 mg). Minimal hypokalaemia may be anticipated at the lower dose, and the other metabolic alterations are less frequently experienced. Moreover, the possibility of

Table 4.21 Drug interactions in antihypertensive therapy

Diuretics

Possible decreased antihypertensive effects

- Cholestyramine and colestipol decrease absorption
- NSAIDs (including aspirin) may antagonize diuretic effectiveness

Possible increased antihypertensive effects

- Thiazide combinations (especially metolazone) with furosemide can produce profound diuresis, natriuresis, and kaliuresis in renal impairment

Effects of diuretics on other drugs

- Diuretics may raise serum lithium levels, thereby increasing toxicity by enhancing proximal tubular lithium reabsorption
- Diuretics may make it more difficult to control dyslipidaemia and diabetes

Beta-blockers

Possible decreased antihypertensive effects

- NSAIDs may reduce beta-blocker effectiveness
- Rifampin, smoking and phenobarbital reduce serum levels of agents

Possible increased antihypertensive effects

- Cimetidine may increase serum beta-blocker levels due to hepatic enzyme inhibition
- Quinidine may promote hypotension

Effects of beta-blockers on other drugs

- Combinations of diltiazem or verapamil may promote additive sinoatrial and atrioventricular node depression and promote negative inotropic effects
- Beta-blockers plus reserpine may promote bradycardia and syncope
- May increase serum theophylline, lidocaine and chlorpromazine levels

Calcium antagonists

Possible decreased antihypertensive effects

- May diminish interactions with rifampin–verapamil; carbamazepine–diltiazem and verapamil; phenobarbital and phenytoin–verapamil

Possible increased antihypertensive effects

- Cimetidine may increase effects of all calcium antagonists

Effects of calcium antagonists on other drugs

- Digoxin and carbamazepine serum levels and toxicity may be increased by verapamil and possibly by diltiazem
- Prazosin, quinidine and theophylline levels may increase with verapamil
- Serum levels of cyclosporine may be increased by diltiazem and nicardipine, and cyclosporine dose may need to be decreased

ACE inhibitors

Possible decreased antihypertensive effects

- NSAIDs (including aspirin) may impair control of blood pressure
- Antacids may decrease ACE inhibitors' bioavailability

Possible increased antihypertensive effects

Effects of ACE inhibitors on other drugs:

- Hyperkalaemia with potassium supplements, potassium-sparing agents and NSAIDs
- ACE inhibitors may increase serum lithium level

ACE, angiotensin-converting enzyme; NSAID, non-steroidal anti-inflammatory drug.

increased total cholesterol and low-density cholesterol levels and, perhaps, lower high-density cholesterol concentration (still a subject of controversy) is less likely to be encountered. In the final analysis, it must remembered that if there is any concern about the metabolic side-effects or any other clinical concern, there are several other alternatives that can be considered. On commencement of diuretic therapy, measurement of these metabolic indices should be made

Table 4.22 Joint National Committee V–VI reports on adverse drug effects

Drugs	*Selected side-effects*	*Precautions and special considerations*
Diuretics		
Thiazide and related agents	Hypokalaemia, hypomagnesaemia, hyponatraemia, hyperuricaemia, hypercalcaemia, hyperglycaemia, hypercholesterolaemia, hypertriglyceridaemia, sexual dysfunction, weakness	Except for metolazone and indapamide, ineffective in renal failure (serum creatinine ≥221 μmol/l [2.5 mg/dl]); hypokalaemia increases digitalis toxicity; may precipitate acute gout
Loop diuretics	Same as for thiazides except loop diuretics do not cause hypercalcaemia	Effective in chronic renal failure
Potassium-sparing agents	Hyperkalaemia	Danger of hyperkalaemia in patients with renal failure and in patients treated with an ACE inhibitor or with NSAIDs
Amiloride		
Spironolactone	Gynaecomastia, mastodynia, menstrual irregularities, diminished libido in males	Renal calculi
Adrenergic inhibitors		
Beta-blockers	Brochospasm, may aggravate peripheral arterial insufficiency, fatigue, insomnia, exacerbation of congestive heart failure, masking of symptoms of hypoglycaemia, hypertriglyceridaemia, decreased high-density lipoprotein cholesterol (except for those drugs with ISA), may reduce exercise tolerance	Should not be used in patients with asthma, (COPD), congestive heart failure with systolic dysfunction, heart block (greater than first degree) and sick sinus syndrome; use with caution in insulin-treated diabetics and patients with peripheral vascular disease; should not be discontinued abruptly in patients with ischaemic heart disease
Alpha–beta blocker Labetalol	Bronchospasm, may aggravate peripheral vascular insufficiency, orthostatic hypertension	Should not be used in patients with asthma, COPD, congestive heart failure, heart block (greater than first degree) and sick sinus syndrome; use with caution in insulin-treated diabetics and patients with peripheral vascular disease
Alpha-1 receptor antagonist	Orthostatic hypotension, syncope, weakness, palpitations, headache	Use cautiously in older patients because of orthostatic hypotension; commonly cough
ACE inhibitors		Rare: angio-oedema, hyperkalaemia rash, ageusia (loss of taste), leukopenia; contraindicated in pregnancy; concerns for hyperkalaemia and aggravation of hypertension in patients with bilateral renal arterial disease or with unilateral disease of a solitary kidney

COPD, chronic obstructive pulmonary disease; ISA, intrinsic sympathomimetic activity.

Table 4.23 Causes for loss of reduced therapeutic responsiveness

- Cost considerations (absolute and copayments)
- Communication
  - Side-effects
  - Dosing instruction
  - Dietary sodium cautions
- Consideration of secondary hypertensions
- Possible need to add a diuretic
  - Atherosclerotic renal arterial disease
  - Symptoms of thyroid disease
  - Primary aldosteronism
  - Exogenous obesity
  - Excessive alcohol intake
  - Other medications

periodically so that therapy might be then modified. Similar considerations should be made with respect to the beta-adrenergic receptor blocking agents or any other agent chosen for initial therapy.

Tables 4.21 and *4.22* describe drug interactions and adverse effects. Some of these problems may be familiar to the practitioner; others are less commonly encountered but are extremely important. Failure (or loss) of responsiveness to antihypertensive therapy is always an important consideration, and may be related to aspects of the professional relationship between the physician and patient (*Table 4.23*).

Further information

National High Blood Pressure Education Program
Office of Prevention, Education, and Control
Department of Health and Human Services
National Insitutes of Health
31 Center Drive
MSC 2480, Building 31
Bethseda, Maryland 20892–2480
USA

Further reading

Frohlich ED: Arthur C. Corcoran Memorial Lecture: Influence of nitric oxide and angiotensin II on renal involvement in hypertension. *Hypertension* 1997;**29**:188–193.

Frohlich ED: Risk mechanisms in hypertensive heart disease. *Hypertension* 1999;**34**:782-78898.

Frohlich ED: Promise of prevention and reversal of target organ involvement in hypertension. *J. Renin Angiotensin Aldosterone Syst.* 2001;**2**(Suppl. 1): S4–S9.

Frohlich ED: Innovative concepts of hypertension to understand and manage the disease. *Med. Clin. N. Am.* 2004;**88**:XIII–XXI.

Frohlich ED: Target organ involvement in hypertension: A realistic promise of prevention and reversal. *Med. Clin. N. Am.* 2004; **88**:209–221.

Frohlich ED: The salt conundrum: A hypothesis. *Hypertension* 2007;**50**:161–167.

Frohlich, ED: Hypertension, In: *Conn's Current Therapy 2007.* Rakel RE, Bope ET, (eds). Saunders Elsevier, Philadelphia 2007, pp. 403–417.

Safar ME, Frohlich ED (eds): *Atherosclerosis, Large Arteries and Cardiovascular Risk.* Karger, Basle, 2007, pp. 117–124.

The Seventh Report of the Joint National Committee on Prevention, Detection, Evaluation, and Treatment of High Blood Pressure (JNC-VII), *JAMA* 2003;**289**:25606–2572.

World Health Organization (WHO)/International Society of Hypertension (ISH) 2003 statement on management of hypertension. World Health Organization, International Society of Hypertension Writing Group. *J. Hypertens.* 2003;**21**:1983–1992.

Zhou X, Matavelli LC, Frohlich ED: Uric acid: Its relationship to renal hemodynamics and the renal renin-angiotensin system. *Curr. Hypertens. Rep.* 2006;**8**:120–124.

Chapter 5

The heart in hypertension

Introduction

A number of cardiac derangements complicate the natural history and progressive course of systemic hypertensive vascular disease. In addition, several independent comorbid diseases, each with its own natural history, can further complicate the overall clinical problem of hypertensive cardiac and vascular disease.

Left ventricular hypertrophy

One cardiac complication of essential hypertension, perhaps the most common, is left ventricular hypertrophy (LVH) (**5.1**). A multiplicity of haemodynamic and non-haemodynamic factors are associated with the development of LVH in essential hypertension (**5.2**).

LVH predisposes the affected patient to microvascular angina pectoris, myocardial ischaemia, interstitial and perivascular fibrosis, apoptosis, infarction, cardiac dysrhythmias, cardiac failure, sudden cardiac death and inflammatory responses (*Table 5.1*). It is exceedingly important for the cardiovascular and primary care physician to recognize the devastating potential of each of those factors as well comorbid diseases that are associated with LVH and hypertensive heart disease. Note that not listed is myocardial infarction resulting from epicardial atherosclerosis, an independent disease with its own natural history and which is exacerbated by hypertension.

The Framingham Heart Study has shown that hypertension is a major risk factor for the development of congestive heart

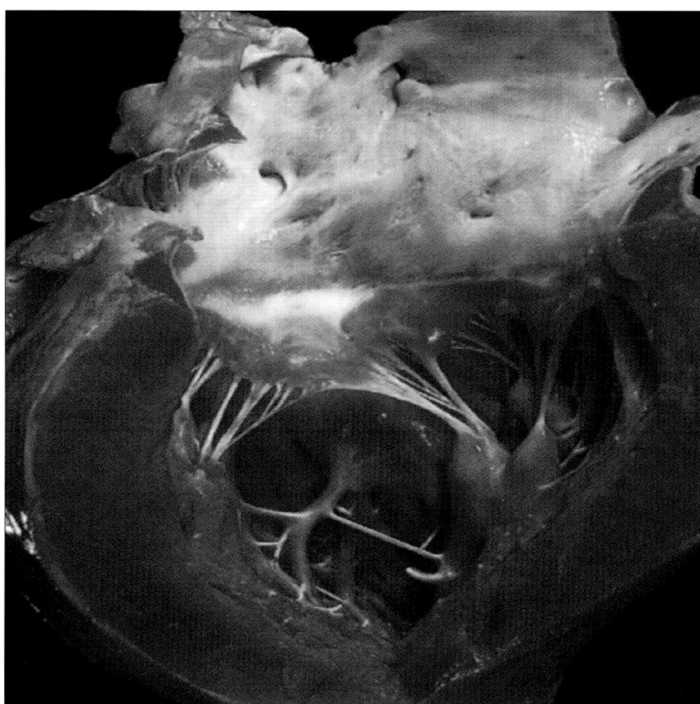

5.1 Left ventricular hypertrophy. Note the marked wall thickening of concentric hypertrophy.

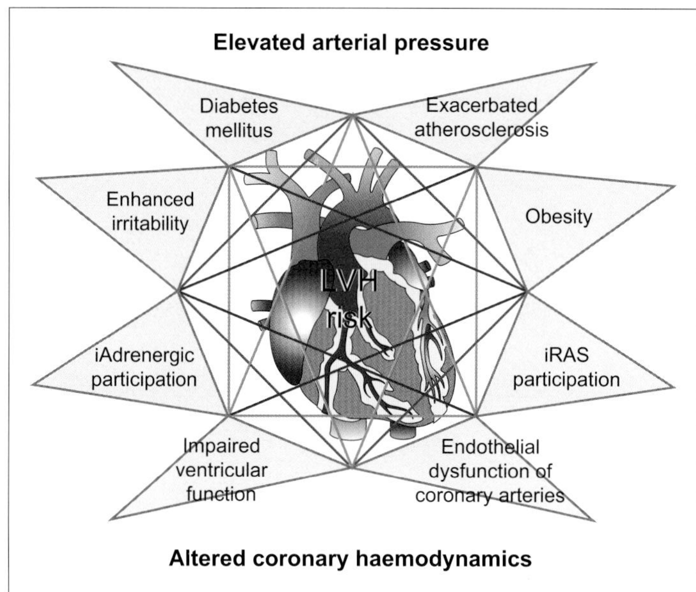

5.2 Mosaic of LVH risk factors showing just some of the factors that contribute to the multifactorial risk associated with LVH.

failure (CHF) (**5.3**). The cumulative incidence of CHF is higher in men than in women and increases with age (**5.4**). In the 1970s systolic heart failure resulting from untreated hypertension was the primary explanation; in the 1990s, diastolic dysfunction, resulting from ischaemia, fibrosis and apoptosis with remodelling, was the main explanation.

Components of hypertensive heart disease and its relationship with atherosclerotic heart disease

Hypertensive heart disease (HHD) is associated with several cardiac and vascular derangements: initiation and progression of LVH; constriction of the coronary arterioles by the same mechanisms that affect the systemic arterioles of all body organs in hypertension; acute and chronic ischaemic hypertensive heart disease with microvascular angina pectoris; endothelial dysfunction of the arterioles and ventricular endothelium; apoptosis; acute and chronic left ventricular failure; ventricular dysrhythmias; and sudden cardiac death. Each of the foregoing alterations increases the likelihood of complications and death from occlusive atherosclerosis of the epicardial coronary arteries.

Atherosclerosis is an independent comorbid disease process that results in occlusion of the larger epicardial coronary arteries and ischaemic disease of the heart, which

Table 5.1 Consequences of LVH in patients with essential hypertension

- Ischaemia
- Ischaemic heart disease
- Coronary artery disease
- Heart failure (systolic/diastolic)
- Remodelling
- Arrhythmias

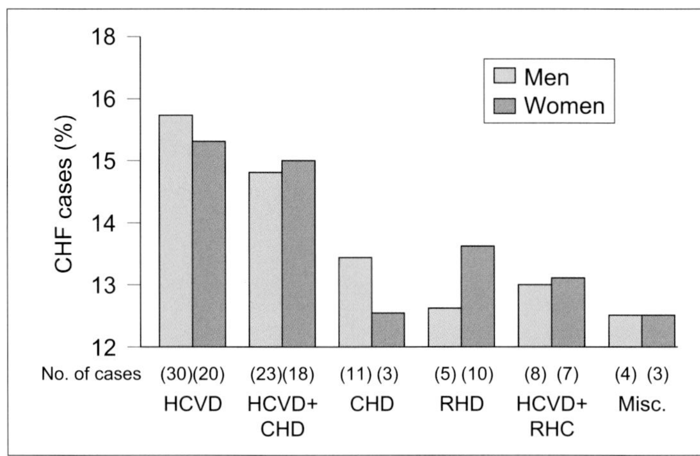

5.3 Causes of congestive heart failure. CHD, coronary heart disease; HCVD, hypertensive cardiovascular disease; RHD, rheumatic heart disease. Reproduced with permission from McKee PA, Castelli WP, McNamara OM, Kannel WB: The natural history of congestive heart failure: the Framingham Heart Study. *N. Engl. J. Med.* 1971;**285**:1795–1801.

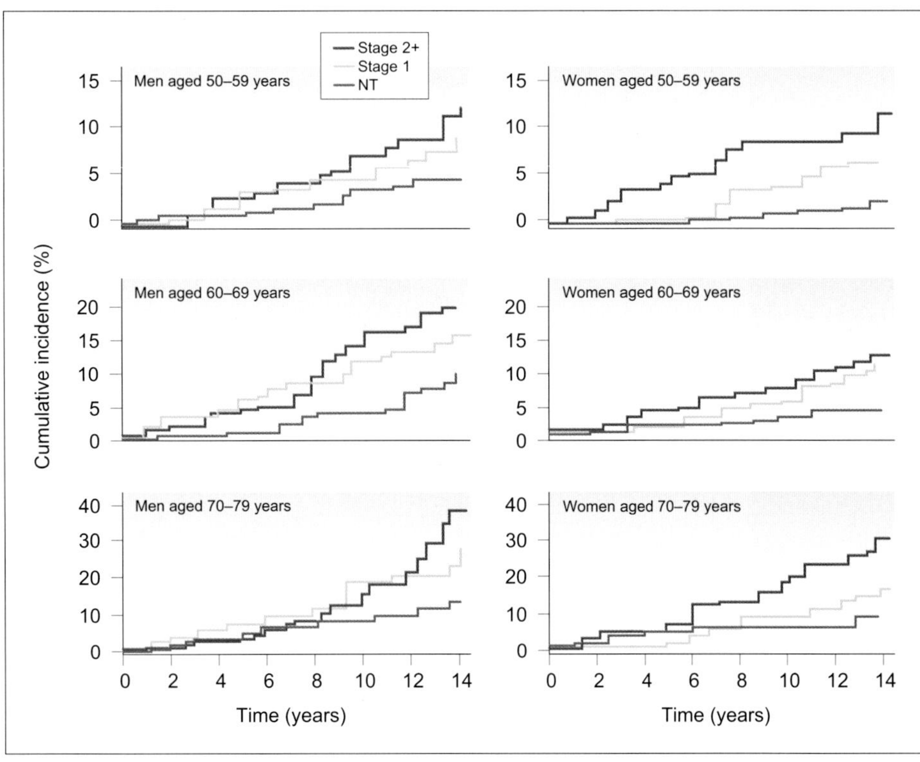

5.4 Cumulative incidence of congestive heart failure by sex and age.

also frequently results in angina pectoris, myocardial ischaemia, fibrosis, infarction, left ventricular failure, cardiac dysrhythmias and sudden cardiac death. Therefore, each of the two diseases, hypertension and atherosclerosis, follows its own natural history (**5.5**), and each accelerates, exacerbates, and is a major underlying risk factor for, the other.

Note that, although the two diseases have similar effects, they differ pathophysiologically. Hypertension is related to increased oxygen demand whereas atherosclerosis relates to insufficient oxygen supply.

Diabetes mellitus

Diabetes mellitus frequently coexists with essential hypertension and may be associated with its own specific cardiac and vascular complications. Diabetes also accelerates and aggravates the development and elaboration of cardiovascular disease (CVD), having its own pathophysiological derangements, which may account for the increased risk for the development of coronary heart disease (CHD). Diabetes is also associated with other cardiac and vascular complications, including those of hypertension. Diabetes impairs tissue perfusion by enhancing the progression of atherosclerotic disease of the medium-sized and larger coronary and other arteries that constitute the microcirculation of the heart, kidneys and other organs. It causes further deterioration of tissue perfusion of kidney, heart, brain, eyes and skeletal muscle that is already impaired by the arteriolar constriction and reduced blood flow and blood flow reserve of these organs as a result of hypertensive vascular disease. In addition, diabetes causes a further degree of enlargement of the left ventricle at any given level of arterial pressure. Whether this is the result of more severe myocardial hypertrophy or of augmented myocardial fibrosis or other infiltrative disease (e.g. protein deposition) remains a subject of intense study.

Note that in the Framingham study patients with diabetes, regardless of gender, developed increased cardiovascular events during follow-up including CHD, heart failure, peripheral vascular disease and stroke (**5.6**).

Glucose intolerance, insulin insensitivity, hypertension, atherosclerosis, hyperlipidaemia and obesity account for a

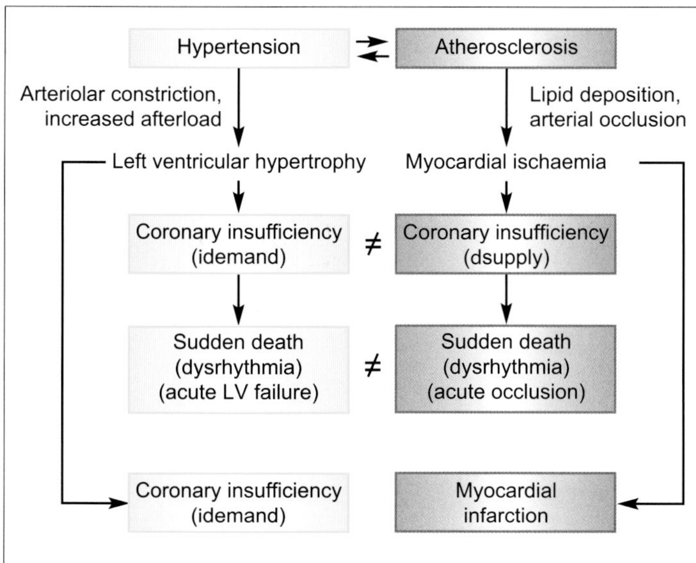

5.5 A general concept detailing the natural history of two cardiac diseases, hypertension and myocardial infarction. Reproduced with permission from Pathophysiology of systemic arterial hypertension Frohlich ED: In: *Hurst's The Heart*, 9th edn. New York, McGraw Hill, 1998, 1635–1650.

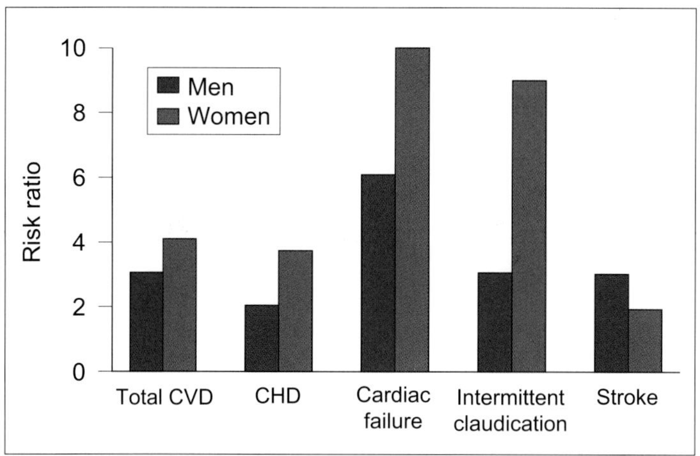

5.6 Framingham Heart Study 30-year follow-up of CVD events in patients aged 35–64 with diabetes ($P < 0.001$ for all values). Reproduced with permission from Wilson PWF, Kannel WB: Epidemiology of hyperglycemia. In: *Hyperglycemia, Diabetes and Vascular Disease.* N Ruderman, J Williamson, N Brownlee (eds). Oxford University Press, New York, 1992, pp. 31–38.

metabolic syndrome (*Table 5.2*), which is of increasing pathophysiological, clinical and therapeutic significance. The prevalence of diabetes has increased markedly in the United States in the last 10 years (**5.7**).

Table 5.2 National Cholesterol Education Program (NCEP) Adult Treatment Panel III (ATP III) criteria for the diagnosis of metabolic syndrome (defined as the presence of three or more of the following factors)

Risk factor	*Defining level*
Abdominal obesity (waist circumference)	
Men	> 40 inches (101 cm)
Women	≥ 35 inches (89 cm)
Triglycerides	≥ 150 mg/dl
High-density lipoprotein cholesterol	
Men	< 40 mg/dl
Women	< < 50 mg/dl
Blood pressure	≥ 130/85 mmHg
Fasting glucose	≥ 10 mg/dl

Obesity

Another disease that commonly coexists with hypertension is *exogenous obesity,* yet another independent risk factor underlying atherosclerosis and CHD. Obesity exacerbates hypertensive heart disease by superimposing a significant volume overload (i.e. preload). The increased venous return to the heart (i.e. cardiopulmonary volume) is superimposed upon the pressure-overloaded left ventricle and expands intravascular volume is in direct proportion to the increase in body mass. Thus, the heart in obese patients with hypertension suffers from volume as well as pressure overload, which, in turn, promotes a dimorphic structural adaptation, one of eccentric as well as concentric LVH.

Other risk factors

Tobacco addiction and hyperlipidaemia are additional independent risk factors underlying coronary heart disease and they also compound the complexity of hypertensive heart disease. Some of these comorbid diseases and complications will be discussed in further detail below. Moreover, other comorbid cardiac diseases may include hypertrophic cardiomyopathy, idiopathic mitral valve prolapse syndrome, myocardial fibrosis or aortic valvular stenosis of the elderly and impaired coronary arterial endothelial dysfunction. And, clearly, the ageing process per se is another complicating factor.

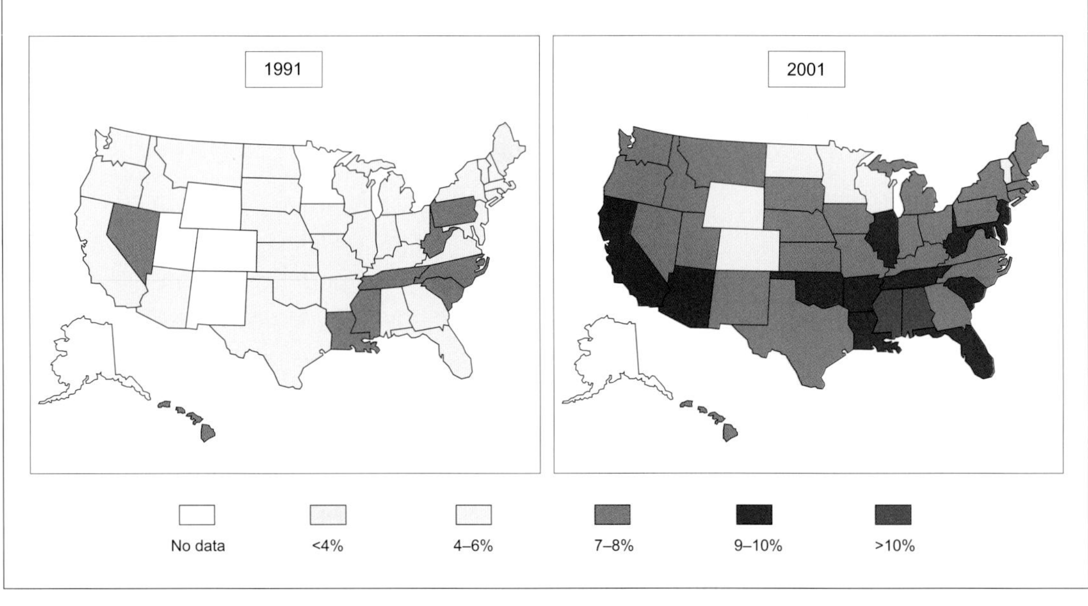

5.7 Prevalence of diabetes in the United States, 1991 and 2001 (national prevalence = 7.9%). Reproduced with permission from Mokdad AH, Ford ES, Bowman BA, Dietz WH, Vinicor F, Bales VS, Marks JS: Prevalence of obesity, diabetes, and obesity-related health risk factors. *JAMA* 2003;**289**:76–79.

Haemodynamic correlates in LVH development

The mass and wall thickness of the left ventricle progressively increase in direct proportion to the unrelenting and progressive afterload imposed upon it by the added chamber stress. In addition, reduced compliance of the aorta and large arteries adds to the effect of afterload imposed on the left ventricle. Thus, although the structural changes of concentric LVH take place in response to the ever-increasing left ventricular afterload, they provide an efficient adaptive means for overcoming the physical forces necessary to maintain stable contractile function. This constitutes a positive aspect of LVH in that it delays the occurrence of left ventricular failure (in the absence of effective antihypertensive therapy). On the other hand, this beneficial feature of LVH is offset by the intrinsic risks of ischaemia, fibrosis, apoptosis and inflammatory responses, which together account for the 'independent' risk of heart failure associated with LVH.

Meerson theory

Felix Meerson suggested several decades ago that the initial response of the heart to pressure overload is the Frank–Starling mechanism, which accounts for ventricular hyperfunction (**5.8**). This functional response results in a period of stable hyperfunction that is associated with the structural adaptation of LVH. Our haemodynamic research work in naturally occurring hypertension has confirmed that the sequence postulated by Meerson occurs in patients with essential hypertension; we further confirmed these findings in the spontaneously hypertensive rat (SHR), which is probably the best experimental model of naturally occurring essential hypertension in humans.

Recent knowledge of LVH development

Recent molecular and cellular biological research has shown that the increased functional performance that results from pressure-overloaded LVH (i.e. the stage of Frank–Starling hyperfunction) is accompanied by a concurrent biological response by the cardiac myocytes. Thus, as the cardiac myocyte is stretched by the initial increase in pressure overload, the cell is stimulated to increase protein synthesis, and cellular hypertrophy results (**5.9**). Thus, the sequence of the cardiac response to pressure overload is not functional followed by structural adaptations; both responses occur simultaneously. The sequence that was postulated earlier by Meerson can now be modified. Instead of the initial hyperfunctional response being followed by structural adaptation, the initial myocytic stretch (induced by pressure overload) evokes simultaneous hyperfunctional and structural adaptive responses. More recent experimental and

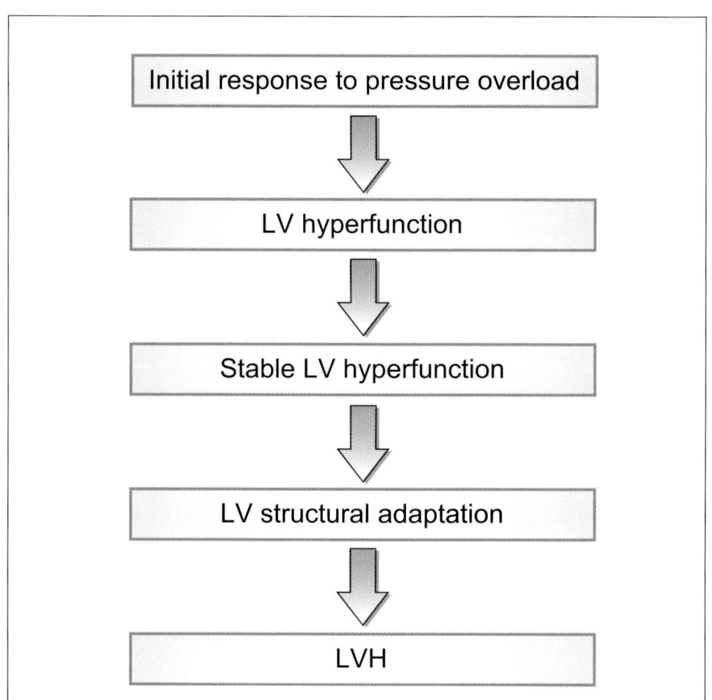

5.8 LVH development according to Meerson.

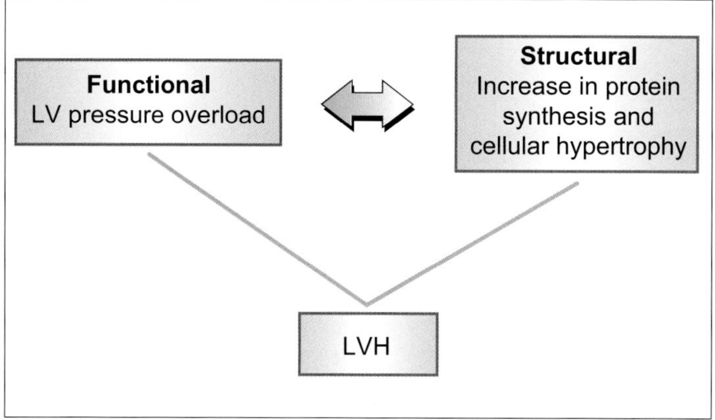

5.9 Recent knowledge of LVH development.

clinical studies have also shown that these structural changes are accompanied by other responses, such as progressive ischaemia (especially on functional demand), extracellular and perivascular fibrosis and enhanced naturally occurring cell death (apoptosis) of the ventricular myocytes, and, probably, inflammatory responses that promote cardiac failure.

Clinical correlates of LVH progression

In our earlier clinical investigative work, we demonstrated that one of the very early changes related to early development of LVH is impaired left ventricular filling during diastole. We have shown that these changes can be identified clinically and electrocardiographically by the presence of an atrial diastolic gallop rhythm (i.e. fourth heart sound or *bruit de gallop*) (see p. 19)(**5.10**, **5.11**). This long-recognized heart sound is a clinical finding that is highly concordant with electrocardiographic indices of left atrial abnormality, higher arterial pressure and an increased prevalence of cardiac dysrhythmias. Indeed, further electrocardiographic studies confirmed our initial findings, enabling us to describe the structural and functional correlates in patients with essential hypertension. In those patients with only left atrial abnormality on ECG, left ventricular mass and septal and posterior wall thickness were increased, associated with the larger left atrium. Furthermore, left ventricular contractility was already impaired at this stage, and those patients with obvious LVH (by ECG) had a significantly larger left ventricle (in terms of mass as well as wall thickness) than those patients with left atrial abnormality only. Moreover, all patients with ECG-apparent LVH exhibited an enlarged left atrium on ECG. Haemodynamically, then, as one progresses from the normal subject to the patient with essential hypertension and atrial enlargement and then to the patient with obvious LVH, arterial pressure and total peripheral resistance increase *pari passu*, and these haemodynamic changes are associated with the structurally adaptive changes of LVH. Furthermore, left atrial enlargement associated with early LVH is accompanied by a reduction in left ventricular ejection rate, and with ECG-apparent LVH the left ventricular ejection fraction becomes impaired. Finally, these ECG correlates were confirmed echocardiographically and it was demonstrated that left atrial abnormality was associated with significant increases in left ventricular mass and wall thickness (**5.12**–**5.14**).

Left ventricular hypertrophy and coronary haemodynamics

In this case not only is the heart affected by LVH, but hypertensive vascular (arteriolar) disease also occurs. Moreover, the disease endpoints are frequently complicated further by improved endothelial function and by coexistent epicardial (atherosclerotic) arterial disease (*Table 5.3*).

Abnormalities of coronary haemodynamics in patients with LVH

More recent clinical investigations have clearly shown that, as LVH progresses, coronary haemodynamics (of both left and right ventricles) also become progressively impaired (*Table 5.4*). Thus, increased total peripheral resistance occurs uniformly in all of the component organ circulations of the systemic circulation, including the coronary arterioles. This increased coronary vascular resistance soon results in a reduction in coronary blood flow and in coronary blood flow reserve. These changes may occur in patients with hypertensive coronary arteriolar disease even in the absence of atherosclerotic occlusive disease of the epicardial

Table 5.3 Hypertensive heart disease

Epicardial arterial disease	*Coronary arteriolar disease*	*Left ventricular hypertrophy*
Endothelial dysfunction	Endothelial dysfunction	Myocytic hypertrophy
Occlusive epicardial	Vasoconstrictor	Ischaemia
Ischaemia	Ischaemia	Collagen deposition
↓Flow reserve	↓Flow reserve	↑Myocardial oxygen demand

Table 5.4 Altered coronary haemodynamics associated with LVF
Structural
Arterial: compression, occlusion, wall thickness
Vessels: reduced in number and density
Left ventricular size: LVH, collagen, protein
Functional
↑Oxygen demand, ↑systolic pressure, ↑left ventricular diameter
Impaired autoregulatory reserve
Endothelial dysfunction
↓NO synthesis
↑Renin–angiotensin system participation
↓Kinin participation

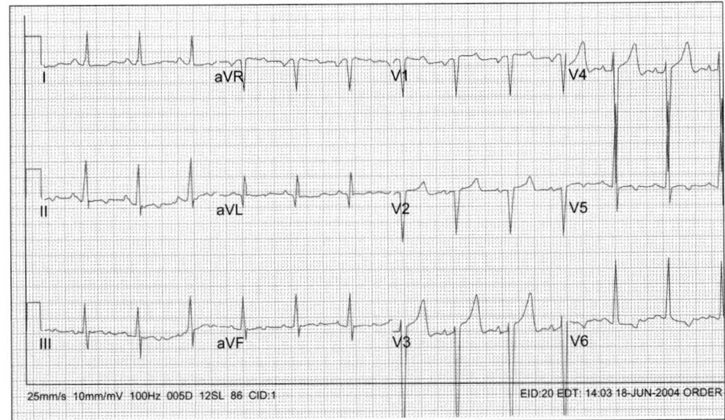

5.10 ECG trace from an asymptomatic patient with LVH. Note the presence of left atrial abnormality (as demonstrated by the increased size of the P-wave and negativity of terminal P-wave changes).

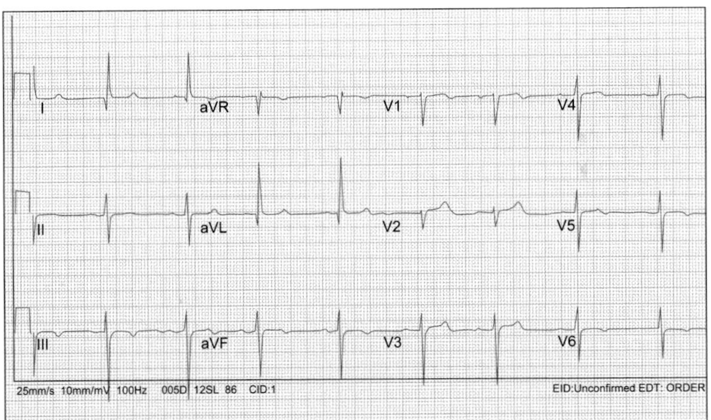

5.11 ECG trace from a patient with LVH showing ST and T changes related to left ventricular strain (LVS). Others have shown arteriographically that coronary blood flow is diminished in patients with LVS.

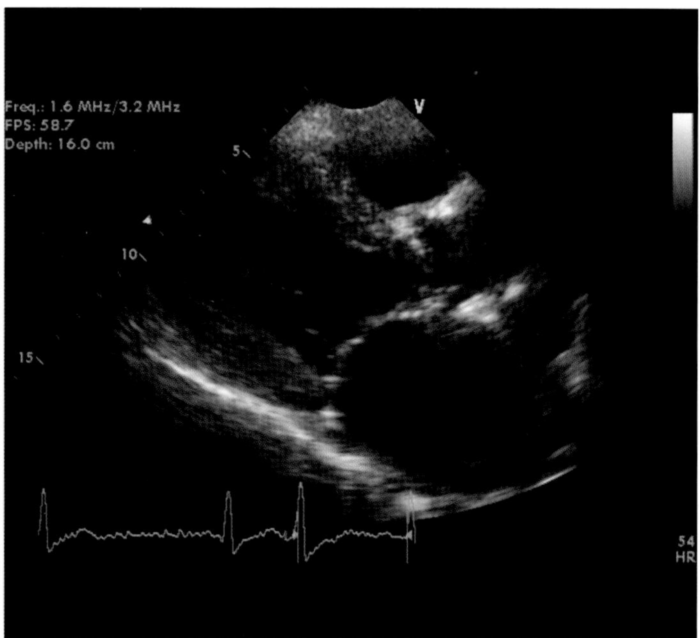

5.12 Two-dimensional echocardiogram from a patient with hypertension demonstrating an increase in left ventricular wall thickness and left ventricular mass and concentric left ventricular hypertrophy.

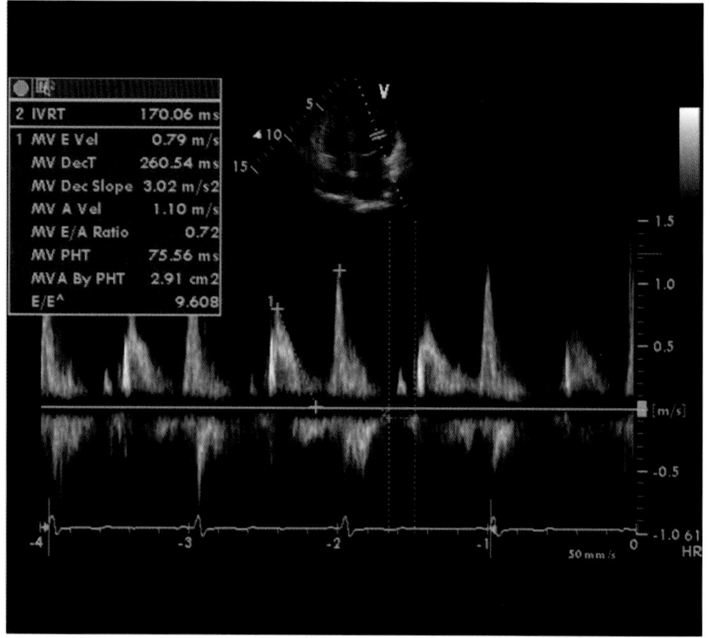

5.13 Doppler echocardiographic image of mitral inflow in a patient with LVH demonstrating relaxation abnormality (abnormal E/A ratio) of the left ventricle.

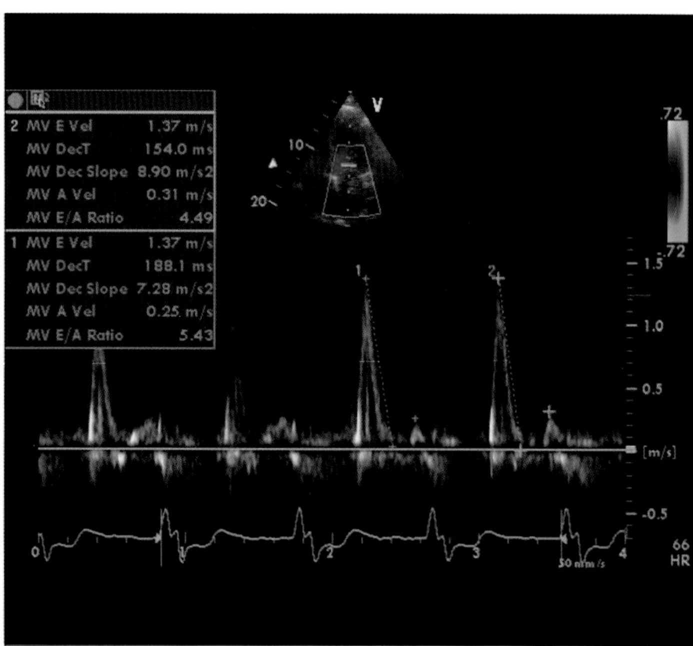

5.14 Doppler echocardiographic image of mitral inflow in a patient with LVH demonstrating diastolic dysfunction (restrictive physiology).

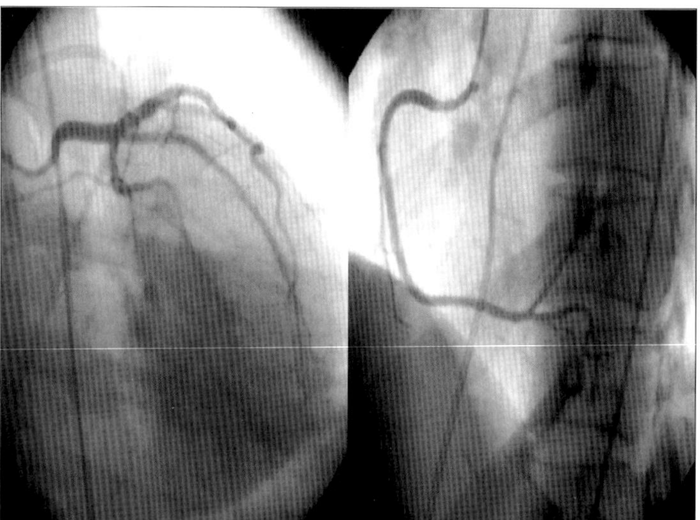

5.15 Coronary angiogram from a patient with hypertension and LVH but without occlusive epicardial coronary artery disease. These findings, then, are consistent with ischaemic heart disease, which may be manifested clinically by 'microvascular angina' and sudden cardiac death, particularly in patients with long-standing hypertension with LVH but without atherosclerosis, in elderly patients and, perhaps, more frequently in women.

coronary arteries (**5.15**). Clearly, however, ischaemic disease of the myocardium is exacerbated when occlusive epicardial coronary atherosclerosis is superimposed upon hypertensive heart disease, especially when LVH is clearly present (**5.16**).

Scheler and colleagues demonstrated this haemodynamic sequence in patients with LVH without ST-segment changes, and then when the LVH was associated with ST-segment deviation during treadmill exercise (**5.17**). Thus, by measuring coronary blood flow before and after administration of the coronary vasodilator dipyridamole, they demonstrated that the LVH is associated with ST-T changes of ischaemia (solid bars) produced by exercise.

Abnormalities in coronary flow and coronary flow reserve in hypertensive rats (SHR) are reversed experimentally towards normal following only 12 weeks' treatment with an angiotensin-converting enzyme (ACE) inhibitor, and to an ever greater extent when ACE inhibitor treatment is combined with angiotensin II (type 1) receptor blocking therapy. In this case, not only is angiotensin II synthesis reduced by ACE inhibitors, but the angiotensin II that escapes inhibition or is inhibited by the ventricular enzyme chimase is antagonized at the type I angiotensin II receptor site (**5.18**).

Non-haemodynamic factors underlying LVH

Over the years it has become apparent that although the development and maintenance of LVH are principally due to haemodynamic factors such as arterial pressure elevation and associated pressure and volume overload, non-haemodynamic factors are also important. Many clinical and experimental studies have provided compelling data to support this thesis. For example, although haemodynamic

5.16 Coronary angiogram from a patient with essential hypertension complicated by occlusive atherosclerotic epicardial coronary artery disease.

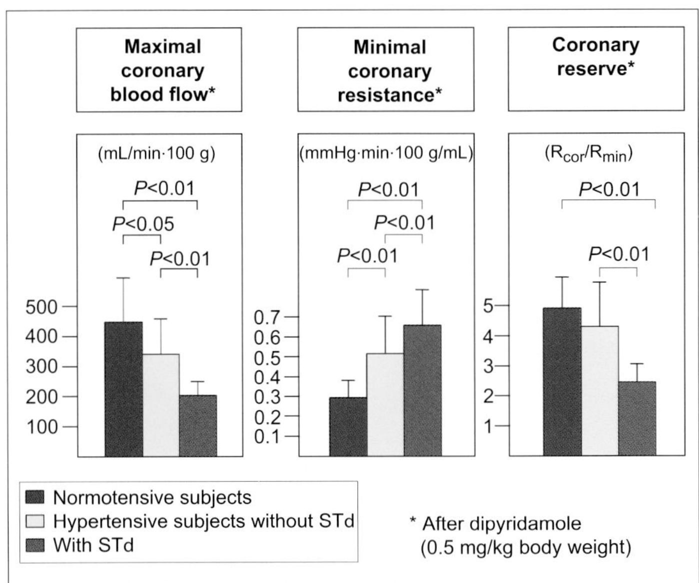

5.17 Coronary blood flow before and after the administration of dipyridamole. Reproduced with permission from Scheler S, Wolfgang M, Strauer BE: Mechanisms of angina pectoris in patients with systemic hypertension and normal epicardial coronary arteries by arteriogram. *Am. J. Cardiol.* 1994;**73**:478–482.

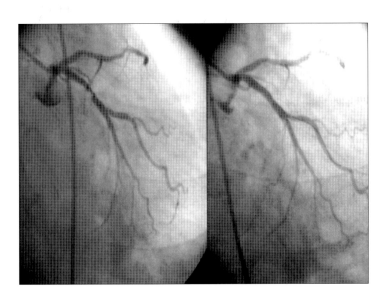

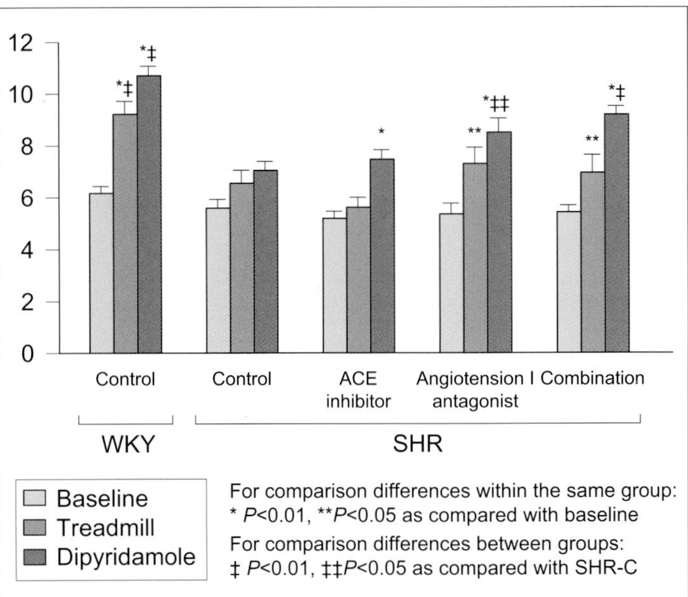

5.18 Left ventricular coronary blood flow and flow reserve.

function has been linked directly to the structural changes of LVH in black patients with hypertension, the association appears to be less in white patients. A similar body of data seems to be accumulating which suggests that development of LVH may be more severe in men than in women (most likely through additional mechanisms). Whether these factors are related to volume, hormonal, humoral or other pressor physiological or growth mechanisms remains a subject of intense investigation and interest at this time.

The foregoing concept is supported by a large body of experimental data. First, there is no clear-cut correlation between increased arterial pressure and left ventricular mass in the experimental model of essential hypertension, i.e. in the spontaneously hypertensive rat (SHR). Moreover, this same functional/structural dissociation has been shown to occur in male and female SHRs treated from conception with beta-adrenergic blocking drugs. Additionally, development of myocardial hypertrophy and increased protein synthesis has been shown when noradrenaline, isoproterenol or angiotensin II is added to myocytes in tissue culture. Further support for this concept is provided by the fact that these agents induce proto-oncogenes, which subsequently leads to cellular protein synthesis. In addition, many classes of antihypertensive agents have been shown to reduce left ventricular mass in non-depressor doses even before arterial pressure is reduced using lower doses of these agents.

Finally, very recent experimental studies in the SHR in our laboratory, as well as clinical studies in men, have shown that salt loading results in cardiac remodelling (with fibrosis) and left ventricular diastolic dysfunction even when arterial pressure is not increased further.

Myocardial fibrosis and collagen deposition

As suggested above, it has been well demonstrated experimentally and clinically that development of pathological LVH is associated with collagen deposition and myocardial fibrosis. Not only is fibrosis of the extracellular matrix and perivascularly in the ventricular wall associated with development and progression of LVH, it also occurs in association with occlusive coronary arterial ischaemic heart disease as well as with the ageing process (**5.20**). These changes are further supported by recent reports that detail the frequency of diastolic dysfunction in experimental hypertension and in patients with hypertension. These changes are exacerbated by further ischaemia associated with epicardial occlusive (atherosclerotic) coronary arterial disease.

Ischaemic changes in the left and right ventricles and fibrosis (demonstrated by hydroxyproline concentration) are associated with ageing in normotensive (WKY) and hypertensive rats (SHR). Note that these changes occur in the right ventricle as well as the left. Hence, pressure overload is not the only factor that accounts for ischaemia and fibrosis (**5.21**).

Fibrosis accompanying LVH, as demonstrated in the experimental studies described above, also occurs in patients with hypertension without atherosclerotic vascular disease. Note that the greater the myocyte diameter

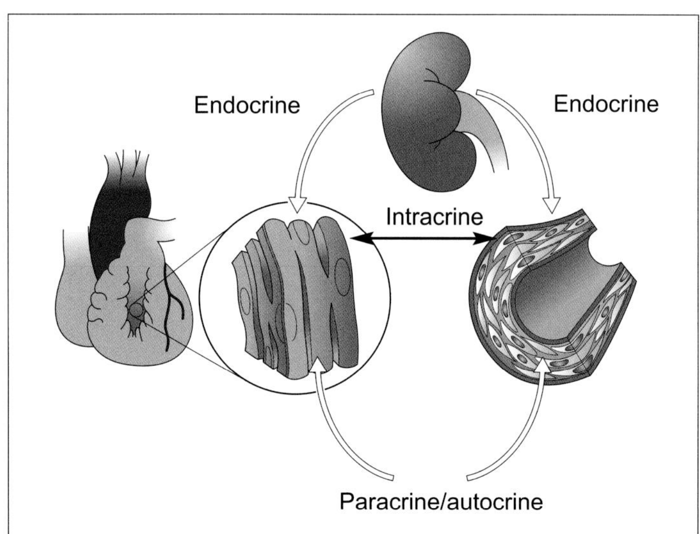

5.19 Systemic and local renin–angiotensin systems.

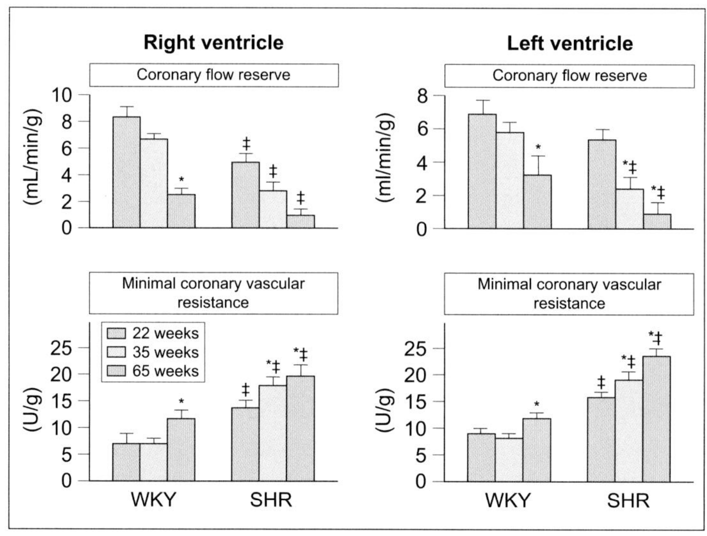

5.20 Ageing and coronary flow reserve.

(hypertrophy), the greater the degree of perivascular and extracellular fibrosis (**5.22**). These changes have been confirmed by endomyocardial biopsy in hypertensive patients without occlusive coronary artery disease by Brilla, Strauer and Diez and their colleagues (see below).

The fibrosis that occurs with progressive LVH has also been demonstrated in patients by Diez and colleagues without performing LV muscle biopsy by measuring circulating procollagen, type I, propeptide in blood (**5.23**).

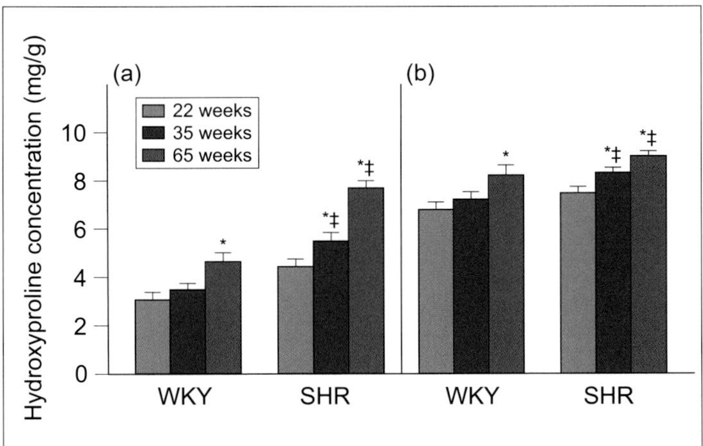

5.21 Ischaemic changes associated with ageing, i.e. fibrosis (determined by concentration of hydroxyproline), in (a) the left and (b) the right ventricles of normotensive (WKY) and hypertensive rats (SHR).

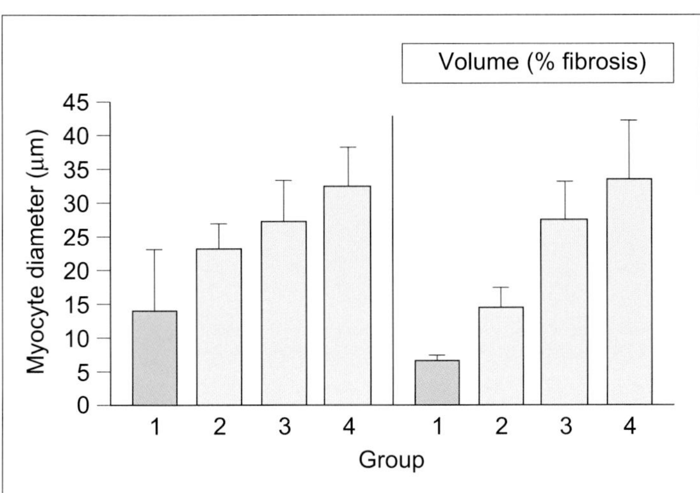

5.22 Pathological fibrosis and connective tissue matrix in human left ventricular hypertrophy. Reproduced with permission from Rossi, MH: Pathologic fibrosis and connective tissue matrix in left ventricular hypertrophy due to chronic hypertension in humans. *J. Hypertens.* 1998;**16**:1031–1041.

Ventricular dysfunction and structural changes

Myocardial ischaemia and fibrosis are manifested clinically by impaired organ function. These effects of LVH were demonstrated many years before effective antihypertensive therapy was available. Systolic function was impaired because severe pressure overload adversely affected the performance of the left ventricle. These patients had no evidence of symptomatic ischaemic myocardial disease, although their systolic contractile function was significantly impaired. More recently, with preserved systolic function, diastolic dysfunction has been found to be the most common expression of cardiac failure in hypertension as well as in elderly patients or patients with ischaemia resulting from atherosclerotic coronary arterial disease. These pathophysiological alterations, whether due to hypertension, ageing or atherosclerotic disease, are all associated with increased ventricular collagen deposition. This, no doubt, adds to the stiffness and reduced distensibility of the ventricular chamber, thereby restricting ventricular filling and contractility.

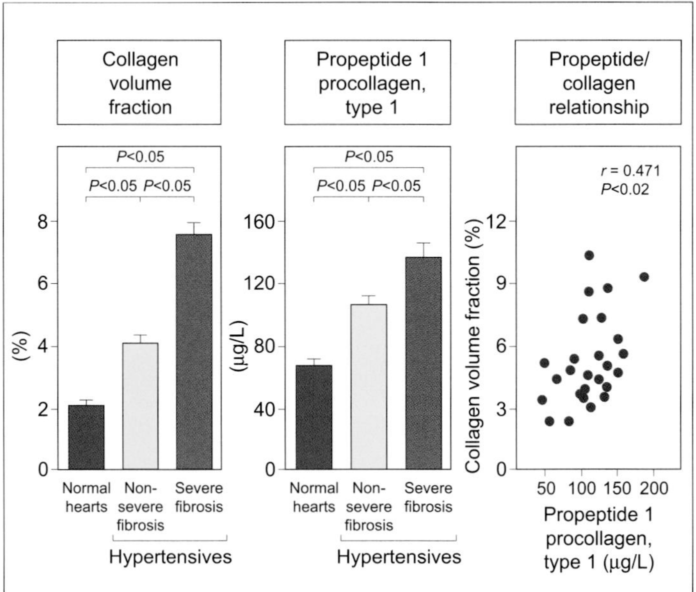

5.23 Plasma–collagen relationships. (a) Collagen volume fraction. (b) Propeptide 1, procollagen, type 1. (c) Propeptide–collagen relationship. Reproduced with permission from Querojota R, Varo N, Lopez B, Larman M, Artinano E, Etayo JC, Diez J: Serum carboxy-terminal propeptide of procollagen type I is a marker of myocardial fibrosis in hypertensive heart disease. *Circulation* 2000;**101**:1729–1735.

Cardiac failure

Note that **5.21**, **5.22** and **5.23** illustrate the alterations associated with diastolic dysfunction, the risk factors associated with development of diastolic heart failure and the similarities and differences between systolic and diastolic heart failure. Moreover, it is important to point out that diastolic heart failure (with preserved systolic function) is the most common cause of hospitalization in patients over 65 years of age in the USA and elsewhere around the world.

Heart failure and antihypertensive therapy

Congestive heart failure can be reduced significantly by antihypertensive therapy. This was first shown in the initial controlled multicentre Veterans Administration Cooperative studies when only hydrochlorothiazide, reserpine and hydralazine were available. With the subsequent introduction of beta blockers, ACE inhibitors, angiotensin II (type 1) receptor blockers and calcium antagonists, it should be quite possible to halt and reverse the increase in hospitalizations that has occurred in the past. However, this has not yet been achieved as currently blood pressure is adequately controlled in only 39% of hypertensive patients. Moreover, treatment today should include more therapy that not only controls pressure, but also improves coronary blood flow reserve and reverses fibrosis and apoptosis. The lesson is clear: we must initiate anti-hypertensive therapy as soon as possible and achieve effective blood pressure reduction. Control is an absolute necessity!

Reversal of hypertrophy

All agents that reduce arterial pressure, if used for long enough, will reduce left ventricular mass and wall thickness and, hence, will reverse LVH. However, certain agents result in a more rapid reversal of LVH (even within 3–12 weeks) in laboratory animals and in hypertensive patients. The rapidity with which LVH can be reduced strongly suggests that certain antihypertensive agents may, as described earlier, possess specific non-haemodynamic qualities that participate in the reversal of LVH and its epiphenomenon. It is now particularly apparent that, in addition to reduction of left ventricular mass and wall thickness, reversal of fibrosis and remodelling and of apoptosis is necessary to reduce the cardiac events associated with LVH.

Left ventricular hypertrophy and stroke

Early multicentre antihypertensive drug trials, whether controlled by placebo or with active controls, demonstrated a significant reduction in fatal and non-fatal strokes (**5.24**). This is because the cerebral circulation is highly pressure dependent.

The Losartan Intervention For Endpoint (LIFE) reduction in hypertension study was a double-blind, randomized, parallel-group trial to compare the effects of losartan and atenolol on cardiovascular morbidity and mortality in 9193 high-risk hypertensive patients (systolic BP 160–200 mmHg or diastolic BP 95–115 mmHg) with LVH determined by electrocardiography (ECG) (**5.25**). The LVH measure used in the study was the product of QRS duration (in ms) and Cornell voltage (the sum of R-wave in AVL plus S-wave in V3 with adjustment of 8 mm in women) using a partition value of >2440 mm × ms (for patients recruited after 30 April 1996 [*n* = 7708], Cornell voltage adjustment was reduced to 6 mm in women, and Sokolow–Lyon voltage of greater than 38 mm was accepted as an alternative measure of the presence of LVH).

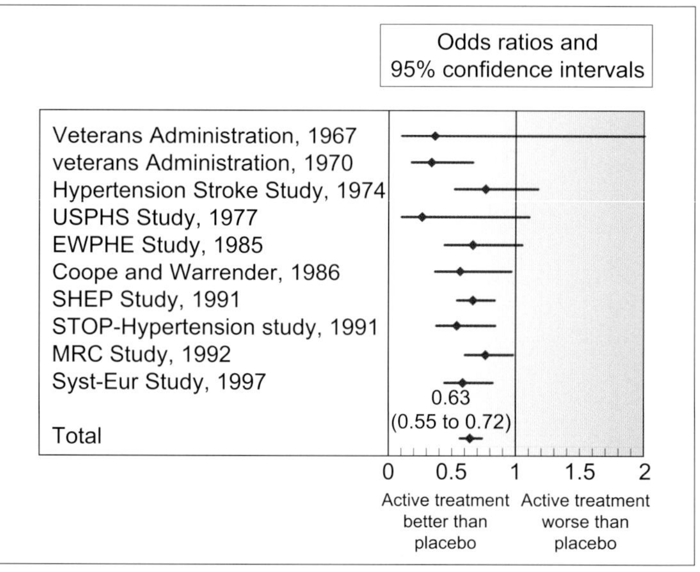

5.24 Relative risk for stroke. From He J, Whelton PA: Elevated systolic blood pressure and risk of cardiovascular and renal disease and randomized controlled trials. *Am. Heart J.* 1999;**138**:211–219.

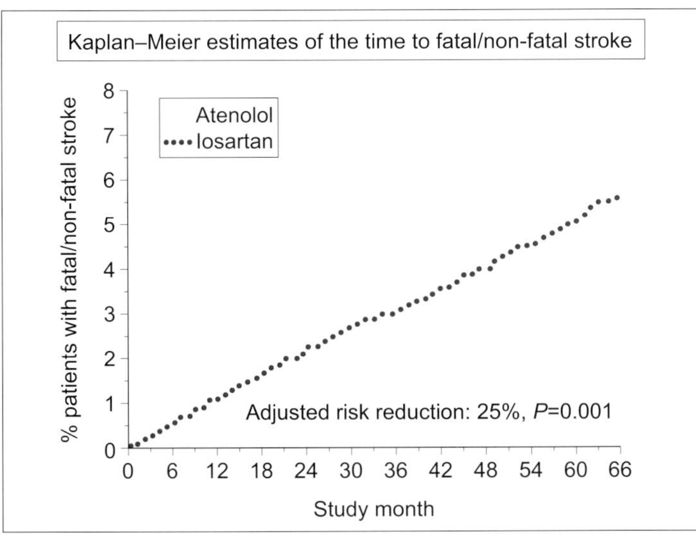

5.25 LIFE: fatal/non-fatal stroke.

Left ventricular hypertrophy and regression of fibrosis

Note that ACE inhibitors as well as a calcium antagonist reduced the concentration of hydroxyproline (thus reducing fibrosis) in the left ventricle in SHRs (**5.26** and **5.27**). The calcium antagonist, however, increased right ventricular collagen, but this was prevented when an ACE inhibitor was added to the calcium antagonist (**5.28**).

Treatment with ACE inhibition for 12 months markedly reduced fibrosis (measured from right septal biopsy) in a patient with LVH and hypertension reported by Strauer and coworkers.

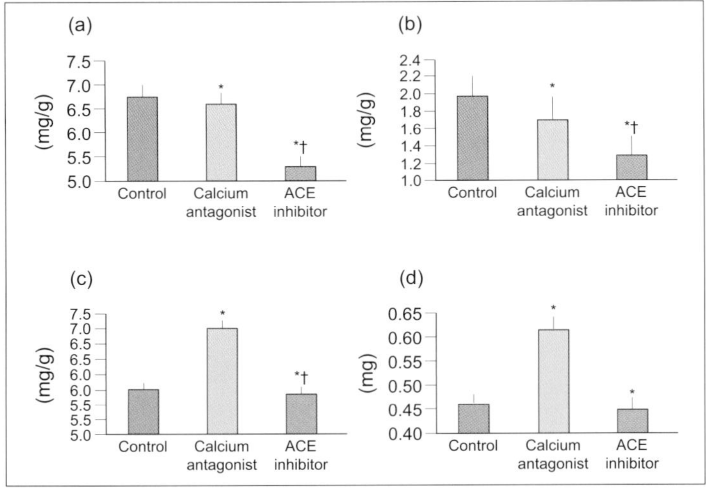

5.26 Myocardial hydroxyproline concentration in 80-week-old SHR. (a) Left ventricular hydroxyproline concentration. (b) Left ventricular hydroxyproline content. (c) Right ventricular hydroxyproline concentration. (d) Right ventricular hydroxyproline content.

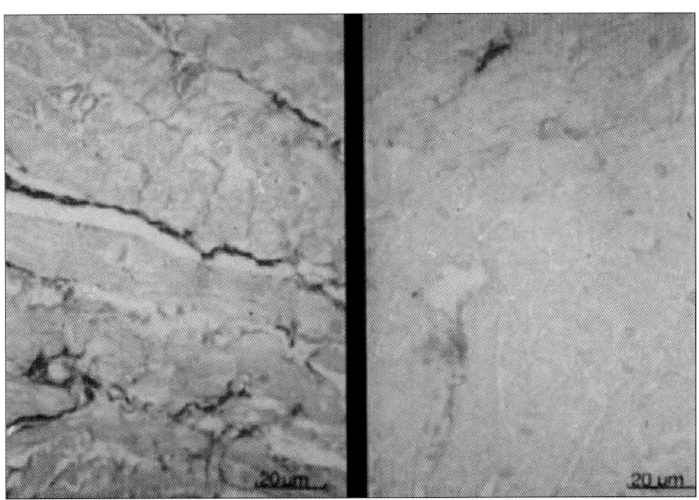

5.27 Right septal biopsy (a) before treatment and (b) 12 months after treatment with ACE inhibition.

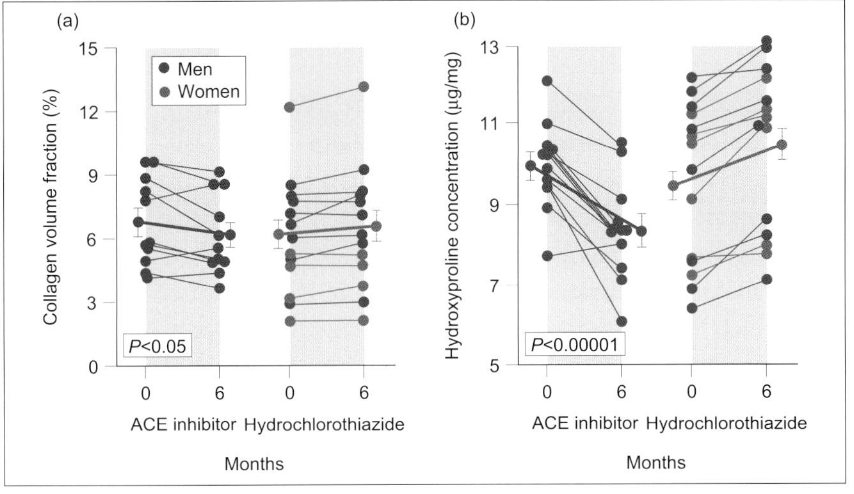

5.28 Myocardial fibrosis in patients treated with either an ACE inhibitor or hydrochlorothiazide as determined by collagen volume fraction (a) or hydroxyproline concentration (b). Reproduced with permission from Brilla CG, Funck RC, Rupp RH: Lisinopril-mediated regression of myocardial fibrosis in patients with hypertensive heart disease. *Circulation* 2000;**102**:1388–1393.

Disparate effects of diuretics and ACE inhibitors on myocardial fibrosis

Note, again, that LV collagen was significantly reduced with ACE inhibitor treatment, but not (increased) with the diuretic hydroclorothiazide (Brilla and colleagues)

Implications of LVH reversal

Patients in whom LVH is reversed by antihypertensive therapy exhibit a lower rate of cardiovascular events on follow-up (**5.29**). Angiotensin receptor blockers but not calcium antagonists reduce the apoptosis (or programmed cell death) index in normotensive patients and patients with hypertension. These data also suggest that the greater amount of apoptosis in patients with hypertension (compared with normotensive subjects) may be a further explanation for the increased prevalence of cardiac failure in hypertension.

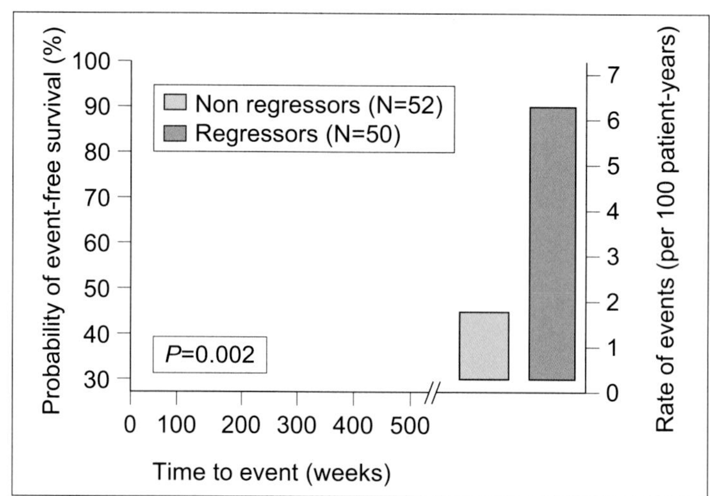

5.29 Reversal of cardiac hypertrophy in hypertensive patients with initial LVH treated by antihypertensive drug therapy. Yellow bar, non-regressors (n = 52); blue bar, regressors (n = 50). Reproduced with permission from Verdecchia P, Schillaci G, Borgioni C, Ciucci A, Gattobiogio R, Zampi I, Reboldi G, Porcellati C: Prognostic significance of serial changes in left ventricular mass in essential hypertension. *Circulation* 1998;**97**:48–54.

Putative mechanisms that explain the reduction in cardiovascular risk with reversal of LVH

1 Reduced arterial pressure.
2 Reduced myocardial oxygen demand.
3 Reduced ventricular fibrosis.
4 Reduced apoptosis.
5 Increased coronary blood flow and flow reserve.
6 Reduced left ventricular mass associated with decreased systolic pressure and decreased cardiac diameter.

Bibliography

Reports of studies that demonstrate the clinical progression of hypertensive heart disease

Basan RS, Levy D: The role of hypertension in the pathogenesis of heart failure. A clinical mechanistic overview. *Arch. Intern. Med.* 1996;**156**:1789–1796.

Dunn FG, Chandraratna P, deCarvalho JGR, Basta LL, Frohlich ED: Pathophysiologic assessment of hypertensive heart disease with echocardiography. *Am. J. Cardiol.* 1977;**39**:789–795.

Frohlich ED, Apstein C, Chobanian AV, Devereux RB, Dustan HP, Dzau V, Fauad-Tarazi F, Horan MJ, Marcus M, Massie B, Pfeffer MA, Re RN, Roccella EJ, Savage D, Shub C: The heart in hypertension. *N. Engl. J. Med.* 1992;**327**:998–1008.

Frohlich ED, Tarazi RC, Dustan HP: Clinical–physiological correlations in the development of hypertensive heart disease. *Circulation* 1971;**44**:446–455.

Frohlich ED: Current issues in hypertension: old questions with new answers and new questions. *Med. Clin. North Am.* 1992;**76**:1043–1056.

Frohlich ED: Is reversal of left ventricular hypertrophy in hypertension beneficial? *Hypertension* 1991;**18**(l):133–138.

Frohlich ED: LVH, cardiac diseases and hypertension: Recent experiences. J. *Am. Coll. Cardiol.* 1989;**14**:1587–1594.

Frohlich ED: Pathophysiology of systemic arterial hypertension. In: *Hurst's The Heart,* 9th edn. RW Alexander, RC Schlant, V Fuster, RA O'Rourke, R Roberts, EH Sonnenbiick (eds). McGraw-Hill, New York, 1998, pp. 1635–1658.

Frohlich ED: The first Irvine H. Page lecture: The mosaic of hypertension: Past, present, and future. *J. Hypertens.* 1988;**6**(Suppl. 4):S2–Sl1.

Frohlich ED: Risk mechanisms in hypertensive heart disease. *Hypertension* 1999;**34**:782–789.

Frohlich ED: Hypertensive heart disease: Time for new paradigms. In: The Local Cardiac Renin-Angiotensin System (Frohlich ED, Re RN eds). Springer, New York, 2005, pp. 1–5.

Komuro 1, Shibazaki Y, Kurabayashi M, Takaku F, Yazaki Y: Molecular cloning of gene sequences from rat heart rapidily responsive to pressure overload. *Circ. Res.* 1990;**66**:979–985.

Pringle SD, Dunn FD, Tweddel AC, Martin W, MacFarlane PW, McKillop JH, Lorimer AR, Cobbe SM, Syjmptomatic and silent myocardial ischemia in hypertensive patients with left ventricular hypertrophy. *Br. Heart J.* 1992;**67**:377–382.

Sokoiow M, Perloff D: Prognosis of essential hypertension treated conservatively. *Circulation* 1961;**33**:87–97.

Major reports dealing with the structural and functional characteristics of left ventricular hypertrophy

Grossman W, Jones D, McLaurin LP: Wall stress and patterns of hypertrophy in the human left ventricle. *J. Clin. Invest.* 1975;**56**:56–64.

Meerson FZ: Compensatory hyperfunction, hyperadaptation, and insufficiency of the heart. *In The Failing Heart. Adaptation and Deadaptation.* AM Katz (ed.). New York, Raven Press, 1983, pp. 47–66.

Important echocardiographic studies that have led to the significance of LVH as a major cardiovascular risk factor

Bikkina M, Levy D, Evans JC, Larson MG, Benjamin EJ, Wolf PA, Castelli WP: Left ventricular mass and the risk of stroke in an elderly cohort: The Framingham Heart Study. *JAMA* 1994;**272**:33–36.

Koren MJ, Devereux RB, Casale PN, Savage DD, Laragh JH: Relation of left ventricular mass and geometry to morbidity and mortality in uncomplicated essential hypertension. *Ann. Intern. Med* 1991;**114**:345–352.

Levy D, Anderson KM, Savage DD, *et al.*: Echocardiographically detected left ventricular hypertrophy: Prevalence and risk factors. The Framingham Heart Study. *Ann. Intern. Med* 1988;**108**:7–13.

Levy D, Garrison RJ, Savage DD, Kannel WB, Castelli WP: Prognostic implications of echocardiographically determined left ventricular mass in The Framingham Heart Study. *N. Engl. J. Med* 1990;**322**:1561–1566.

Levy D, Larson MG, Vasan RS, Kannel WB, Ho KKL: The progression from hypertension to congestive heart failure. *JAMA* 1996;**275**:1557–1562.

Levy D, Salomon M, D'Agostino RB, Belanger AJ, Kannel WB: Prognostic implications of baseline electrocardiographic features and their serial changes in subjects with left ventricular hypertrophy. *Circulation* 1994;**90**:1786–1793.

Sheps S, Frohlich ED: Limited echocardiography for hypertensive left ventricular hypertrophy. *Hypertension* 1997;**29**:519–524.

Reports that have suggested non-haemodynamic factors are important in the development and reversal of LVH

Frohlich ED, Tarazi RC: Is arterial pressure the sole factor responsible for hypertensive cardiac hypertrophy? *Am. J. Cardiol* 1979;**44**:959–963.

Frohlich ED: Is reversal of left ventricular hypertrophy in hypertension beneficial? *Hypertension* 1991;**18**(l):133–138.

Reports emphasizing role of collagen and hormonal factors in development and reversal of LVH

Arita M, Horinaka S, Frohlich ED: Biochemical components and myocardial performance after reversal of left ventricular hypertrophy in spontaneously hypertensive rats. *J. Hypertens.* 1993;**11**:951–959.

Morgan HE, Baker KM: Cardiac hypertrophy: mechanical, neural, and endocrine dependence. *Circulation* 1991;**83**:13–25.

Tarazi RC, Frohlich ED: Is reversal of cardiac hypertrophy a desirable goal of antihypertensive therapy? *Circulation* 1987;**75**(1):113–117.

Weber KT, Anverson P, Armstrong PW, Brilla CG, Burnett JC Jr. Cruickshank JM, Devereux RB, Giles TD, Korsgaardn, Leier CV, Mendelsohn FAO, Motz WH, Mulvany MI, Strauer BE: Remodeling and reparation of the cardiovascular system. *J. Am. Coll. Cardiol.* 1992;**20**:3–16.

Weber KT, Brilla CG: Pathological hypertrophy and cardiac interstitium. Fibrosis and renin- angiotensin-aldosterone system. *Circulation* 1991;**83**:1849–1865.

Weber KT, Sun Y, Guarda E: Structural remodeling in hypertensive heart disease and the role of hormones. *Hypertension* 1994;**23**:869–877.

Weber KT: Editorial. Monitoring tissue repair and fibrosis from a distance. *Circulation* 1997;**96**:2488–2492.

Reports relating coronary flow in LVH and its reversal

Houghton JL, Frank Mj, Carr AA, et al: Relations among impaired coronary flow reserve, left ventricular hypertrophy and thallium perfusion defects in hypertensive patients without obstructive coronary artery disease. *J. Am. Coll. Cardiol.* 1990; **15**:43–51.

Marcus ML, Harrison DG, Chilian WM, et al: Alterations in the coronary circulation in hypertrophied ventricles. *Circulation* 1987;**75**(l):19–25.

Nunez E, Hosoya H, Susic D, Frohlich ED: Enalapril and losartan reduced cardiac mass and improved coronary hemodynamics in SHR. *Hypertension* 1997;**29**:519–524.

Scheler S, Wolfgang M, Strauer BE: Mechanisms of angina pectoris in patients with systemic hypertension and normal epicardial coronary arteries by arteriogram. *Am. J. Cardiol.* 1994;**73**:478–482.

Susic D, Nunez E, Hosoya H, Frohlich ED: Coronary hemodynamics in aging spontaneously hypertensive and normotensive Wistar-Kyoto rats. *J. Hypertens.* 1998;**16**:231–237.

Studies emphasizing importance of impaired endothelium-dependent vasodilatation in patients with hypertension

Frohlich ED: *1996* Arthur C. Corcoran Lecture: Influence of nitric oxide and angiotensin 11 on renal involvement in hypertension. *Hypertension* 1997;**2**:188–193.

Gerhard M, Roddy MA, Creager Sj, Creager MA: Aging progressively impairs endothelium- dependent vasodilation in forearm resistance vessels of humans. *Hypertension* 1996;**27**:849–853.

Panza JA, Garcia CE, Kilcoyne CM, Quyyumi AA, Cannon RO III: Impaired endothelium-dependent vasodilation in patients with essential hypertension. Evidence that nitric oxide abnormality is not localized to a single signal transduction pathway. *Circulation* 1995;**91**:1732–1738.

Treasure CB, Klein JC, Vita JA, Manoukianu SV, Renwixh GH, Selwyn AP, Ganz P, Alexander RW: Hypertension and left ventricular hypertrophy are associated with impaired endothelium-mediated relaxation in human coronary artery resistance vessels. *Circulation* 1993;**87**:86–93.

Reports suggesting the participation of the J-shaped curve phenomenon in hypertension and myocardial infarction

Collins C, Peto R. MacMahon S. Hebert H, Hebach NH, Eberlein KA, Godwin J, Olzilbash N, Taylor JO, Hennekens CH: Blood pressure, stroke and coronary heart disease. Part *2.* Short-term reductions in blood pressure overview of randomised drug trials in their epidemiological context. *Lancet* 1990;**335**:827–838.

Cruickshank JM, Thorp JM, Zacharias Fj: Benefits and potential harm of lowering high blood pressure. *Lancet* 1987;**1**:581–584.

Cruickshank JM: Coronary flow reserve and the J-curve relation between diastolic blood pressure and myocardial infarction. *BMJ* 1988;**297**:1227–1230.

MacMahon S, Peto R, Cutler J, Collins R, Sorlie P, Neaton J, Abbott R, Godwin J, Dyer A, Stamlerj: Blood pressure, stroke, and coronary heart disease. Part 1. Prolonged differences in blood pressure: Prospective observational studies corrected for the regression dilution bias. *Lancet* 1990;**335**:765–774.

Thijs L, Fagard R, Lijnen P, Staessen J, VanHoot R, Amery A: A meta-analysis of outcome trials in elderly hypertensives. *J. Hypertens.* 1992;**10**:1103–1109.

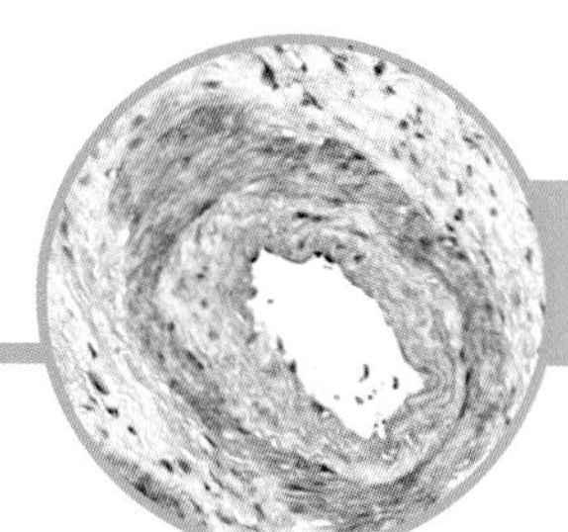

Chapter 6

The kidney in hypertension

Renal parenchymal involvement in hypertension

In contrast to the remarkable reduction in deaths from stroke and coronary heart disease (CHD) that has been achieved primarily as a result of improved control of hypertension (**6.1**), the prevalence of end-stage renal disease (ESRD) in patients with hypertension increases unabated (**6.2**). Some have ascribed this phenomenon to the remarkably increased prevalence of diabetes mellitus and obesity. In part, it reflects broader defined limits to abnormal glucose levels and carbohydrate tolerance as well as for overweight/obesity. But we must also take cognizance of the fact that the incidence of hypertensive disease in patients with diabetes mellitus is extremely high.

Hypertension is extremely common in the general population of acculturated societies (prevalence over 20%), but is much higher in blacks (about 40%) and in the elderly

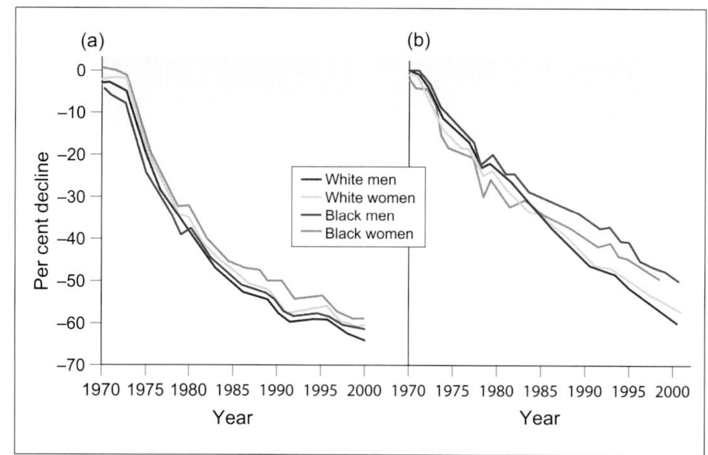

6.1 Reduction in age-adjusted mortality rates for (a) stroke and (b) coronary heart disease by gender and race in the United States.

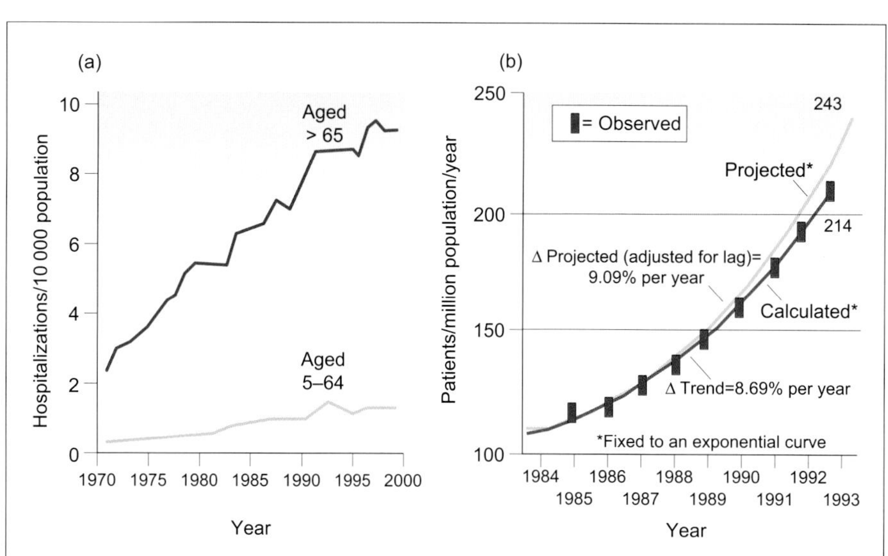

6.2 (a) Hospitalization rates for congestive heart failure and (b) observed and projected treated incidence rates for end-stage renal disease (ESRD) in the United States.

(50% or more). Consequently, hypertensive disease is extremely common in patients with both diabetes and hypertension and is probably even more common in black and elderly patients with diabetes. Even in the early 1920s, when the association of hypertension and diabetes was first reported, hypertensive disease was clearly demonstrated in 50–60% of patients with hypertension over the age of 50 years. This co-occurrence is still extremely common today (> 50%), even with the use of more expanded definitions (or criteria) for hypertension, diabetes mellitus and obesity (alone and/or their mutual coexistence). The point is not to denigrate the popular emphasis on these strong and close relationships, but simply to point out that antihypertensive therapy has not yet led to a reduction in the complication of ESRD as dramatic as the reduction achieved in death rates from stroke and CHD.

Thus, it may legitimately be asked why the prevalence of ESRD continues to increase and why target organ involvement of the kidney has not been reduced by antihypertensive treatment. Various explanations have been proposed (**6.3**).

Table 6.1 Pathophysiological mechanisms favouring development of ESRD in hypertension and diabetes

- Renal ischaemia
- Glomerular sclerosis
- Renal arterial constriction
- Arteriolar hyalinosis
- Glomerular arteriolar constriction
- Intravascular thromboses
- Increased glomerular hydrostatic pressure
- Glomerular hyperfiltration
- Interstitial inflammatory responses
- Others

Despite the fact that antihypertensive therapy has failed to halt the increase in prevalence of ESRD, several well-controlled multicentre trials have shown that reducing target blood pressure in patients with diabetes results in improved renal outcomes. Consequently, all national and international guidelines now recommend that treatment should aim to reduce arterial blood pressure to < 130 and < 80 mmHg (systolic and diastolic, respectively) in all patients with diabetes mellitus or with hypertension-associated renal parenchymal functional involvement, as soon as this becomes apparent. Despite this, there remains no adequate explanation for the continued increase in ESRD.

Several major pathophysiological alterations have been proposed to explain the underlying mechanisms of hypertensive vascular disease or of diabetes mellitus that favour the development of ESRD (*Table 6.1*). These alterations are extremely common in patients with hypertension and/or with diabetes mellitus as well as in elderly normotensive or even non-diabetic patients. Therefore, it is clear that ageing is one major factor that is associated with renal functional impairment not only in patients with hypertension or diabetes mellitus, but also in those who are otherwise normal.

Pathophysiological changes

The renal vasculature is extremely vulnerable to increases in arterial pressure, particularly as a consequence of systemic arterial as well as glomerular arteriolar vasoconstriction. Initially, the afferent glomerular arterioles become more prominently constricted but, as the disease progresses and as arterial pressure increases further, the efferent glomerular arterioles also become progressively constricted. Associated with this renal arterial and glomerular arteriolar constriction, the walls of the intrarenal and glomerular vessels

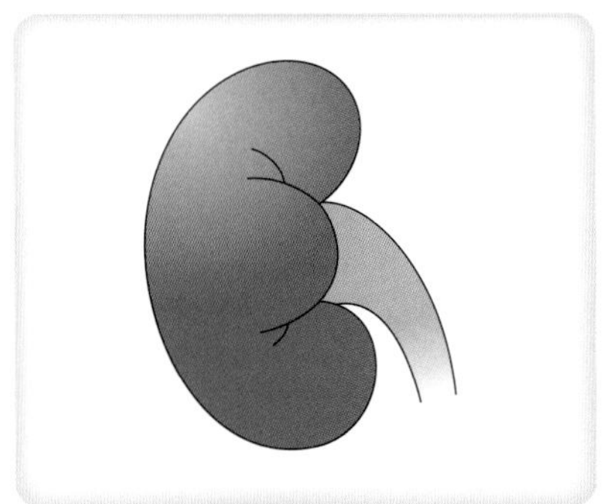

1. Pressures not adequately reduced
2. Renal involvement not reversible by treatment
3. Antihypertensive agents not effective

6.3 Reasons why, of target organ involvement in hypertension, that of the kidney is not reduced by treatment. I favour none of these; but arguments presented herein offer other ideas.

undergo hyaline degeneration, develop progressive sclerosis and thicken. These changes add further to the effects of luminal narrowing and glomerular injury (**6.4**).

Clinical estimates of intrarenal haemodynamic alterations initially utilized the Gomez formulae, which combine measurements of renal plasma flow, glomerular filtration rate, haematocrit and plasma protein concentration. However, with the subsequent introduction of renal micropuncture techniques, studies involving experimental animals with various models of hypertension or diabetes provided more direct measurements of the renal haemodynamic and glomerular dynamic alterations. These techniques have been employed in rats with naturally developing genetic hypertension, so-called spontaneously hypertensive rats (SHRs), and in their normotensive Wistar–Kyoto controls (WKY).

It was found that ESRD develops naturally with ageing (73 weeks) in SHRs, and the findings confirm the earlier pathophysiological changes described in other experimental models (which required more complex interventions with the kidney, the addition of chemicals and drugs, etc.) as well as more indirect measurements in humans. Thus, as mean arterial pressure (MAP) rises, and as afferent and efferent arteriolar constriction progressively increase, the estimated total renal blood flow (ERBF), glomerular filtration rate (GFR) and their ratio, the renal filtration fraction (FF), diminish (**6.5**).

Consequently, the single-nephron plasma flow (SNPF), single-nephron glomerular filtration rate (SNGFR) and single-nephron filtration fraction (SNFF) diminish as a result of the coincident increases in renal afferent (RA) and efferent (RE) resistance and glomerular arteriolar resistance.

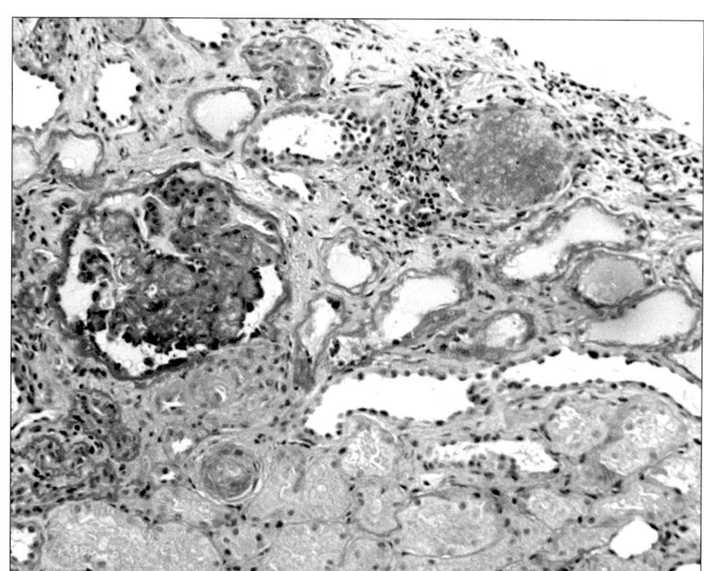

6.4 Renal micrograph demonstrating benign nephrosclerotic changes of the glomerulus and arteriole. Note the hyalinized glomerulus and enlarged segmental sclerotic glomerulus with tubular atrophy and chronic inflammation. Arteriolosclerosis with luminal narrowing of afferent arteriole can be seen.

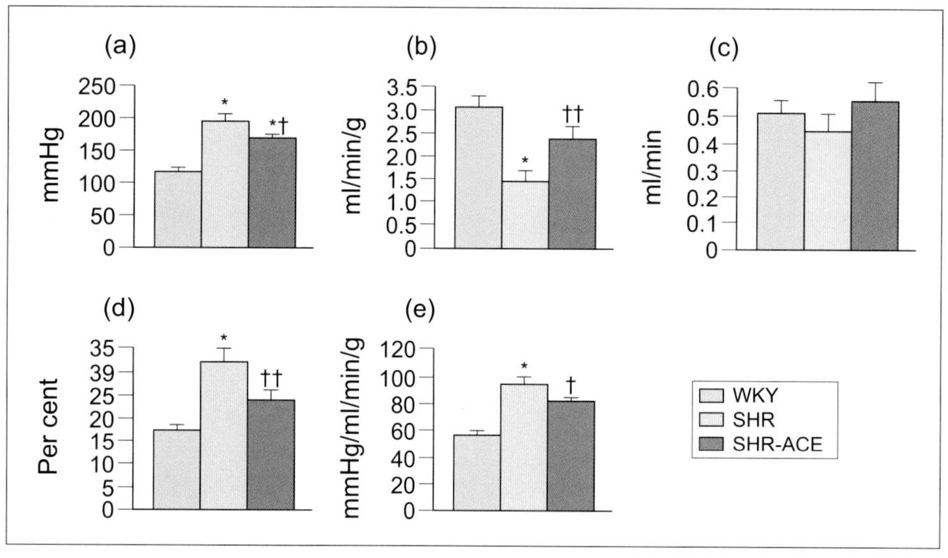

6.5 Haemodynamics and renal function in spontaneously hypertensive rats (SHRs) with naturally developing end-stage renal disease, control Wistar–Kyoto rats (WKY) and SHRs treated with an angiotensin-converting enzyme inhibitor (ACE). (a) Mean arterial pressure. (b) Estimated renal plasma flow. (c) Glomerular filtration rate. (d) Filtration fraction. (e) Renal vascular resistance. $^*P < 0.01$ compared with Wistar–Kyoto rats. $\dagger P < 0.01$, $\dagger\dagger P < 0.05$ compared with SHRs.

These altered glomerular dynamics result in increased intraglomerular arteriolar pressure (RG) and increased hyperfiltration and FF. These changes favour the pathological changes associated with ischaemia and ultrafiltration and result in the leakage of plasma components across the matrix production by vascular smooth muscle cells glomerular capillaries and also, probably, from the intrarenal vasculature into the renal interstitium (**6.6**).

Renal histological studies in 73-week-old SHRs suggest that the severe nephrosclerosis that naturally develops in this model is very similar to that observed more indirectly (using the Gomez formulae) in patients with essential hypertension and ESRD. This suggests that the Gomez formulae are a valid tool and, indeed, these formulae have been used to demonstrate the long-term efficacy of the calcium antagonist diltiazem in patients with arterial disease attributable to essential hypertension (**6.7** and **6.8**).

The results of micropuncture measurements are very closely correlated with the microscopic findings of severe arteriolar and glomerular injury in SHRs and with similarly obtained data from normotensive WKY rats utilizing the arteriolar and glomerular injury scoring criteria of L. Raij and his associates (*Table 6.2* and **6.9**).

Remarkably, and most impressively, when these 73-week-old SHRs were treated for only 3 weeks with an angiotensin-converting enzyme (ACE) inhibitor, the abnormal patho-

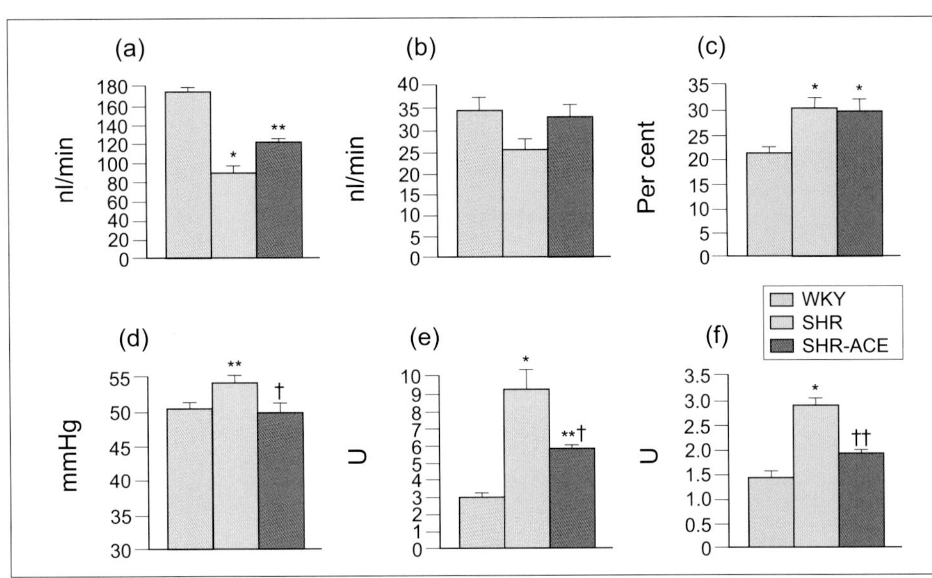

6.6 Glomerular dynamics in naturally developing end-stage renal disease in aged spontaneously hypertensive rats (SHRs), control Wistar–Kyoto rats (WKY) and SHRs treated with an angiotensin-converting enzyme inhibitor (ACE) obtained by renal micropuncture. (a) Single-nephron plasma flow. (b) Single-nephron glomerular filtration rate. (c) Single-nephron filtration fraction. (d) Intraglomerular arterial pressure. (e) Afferent resistance. (f) Efferent resistance. *$P < 0.01$, **$P < 0.05$ compared with Wistar–Kyoto rats. †$P < 0.01$, ††$P < 0.05$ compared with SHRs.

Table 6.2 Glomerular and arteriolar injury scoring

Glomerular		
1	Normal	
2–3	One-third to two-thirds	Focal sclerosis and/or hyalinosis
4	Total	
Arteriolar		
1	Normal	
2–3	< 50%, > 50%	Hyalinosis
4	Total	

Reproduced with permission from Raij L, Azar S, Keane W: Mesangial immune injury, hypertension, and progressive glomerular damage in Dahl rats. *Kidney Int.* 1984;**26**:137–143.

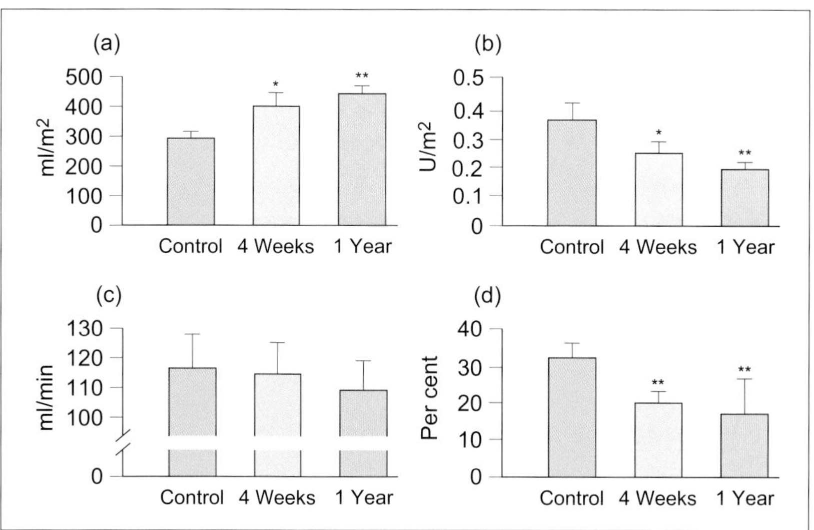

6.7 The renal haemodynamic effects of prolonged diltiazem (300 mg/day) before and 4 weeks and then 1 year after initiation of therapy. (a) Renal blood flow index. (b) Renal vascular resistance. (c) Glomerular filtration rate. (d) Filtration fraction.

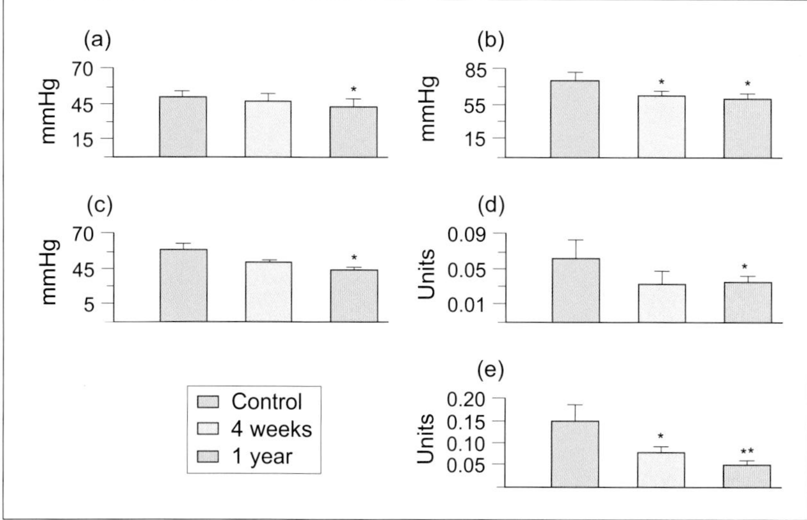

6.8 Calculated glomerular dynamic effects before and 4 weeks and 1 year after initiation of prolonged diltiazem therapy (300 mg/day) therapy. (a) Afferent preglomerular arteriolar pressure. (b) Capillary glomerular pressure. (c) Efferent postglomerular arteriolar pressure. (d) Afferent preglomerular arteriolar resistance. (e) Efferent postglomerular arteriolar resistance.

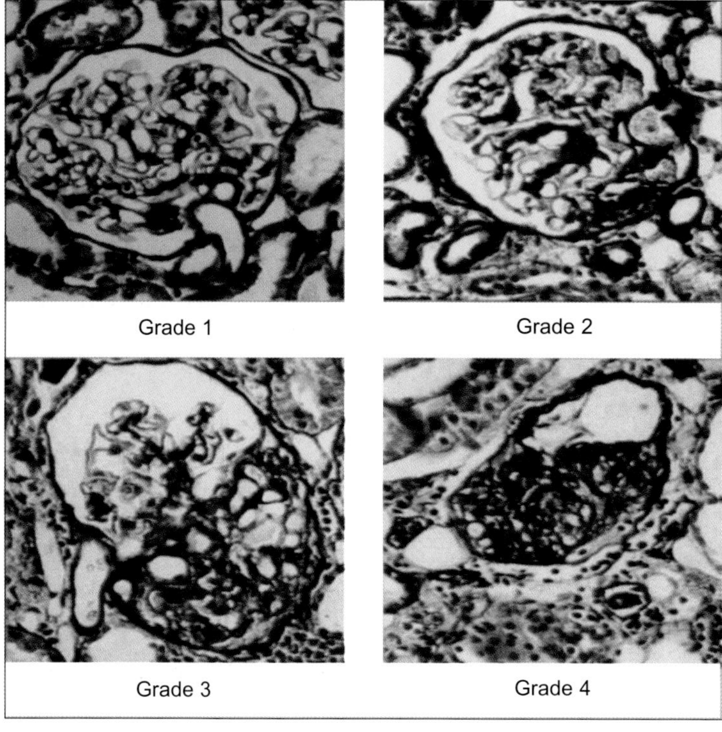

6.9 Micrographs typical of glomerular and arteriolar involvement of the kidney grades 1–4.

physiological measurements obtained by micropuncture were dramatically reversed (**6.10**). Furthermore, these pathological changes were accompanied by a significant reduction in proteinuria (**6.11**). Thus, although the physiological measurements obtained by micropuncture were obtained from the superficial glomeruli with minimal pathological changes (i.e. from less diseased nephrons), the significant (parallel) changes confirm the findings from histological studies of sections of the juxtamedullary glomeruli that cannot be reached by micropuncture in the deeper tissues of the kidney (**6.12**).

Thus, fibrinoid necrosis of the arterioles results as a consequence of the haemodynamic and glomerular dynamic alterations described above and, when the development of

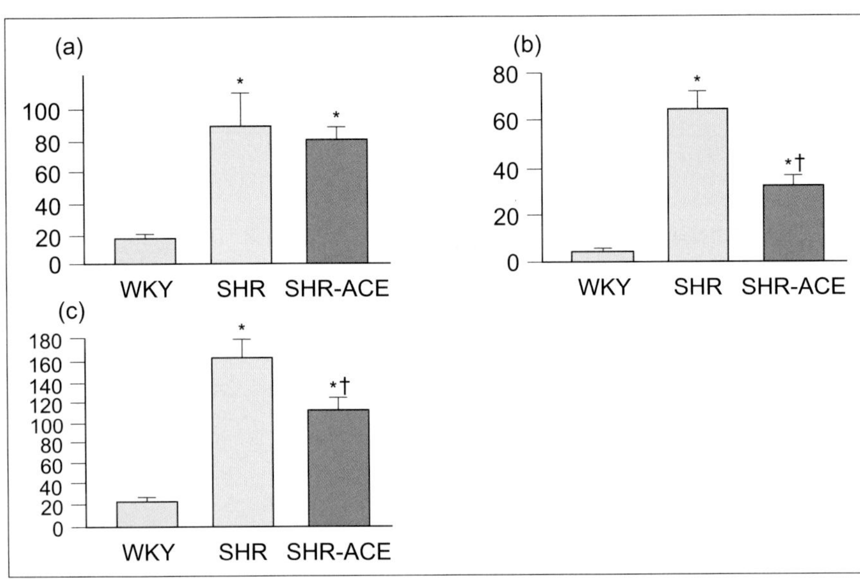

6.10 Glomerular and arteriolar scoring in spontaneously hypertensive rats (SHRs), control Wistar–Kyoto rats (WKY) and SHRs treated with the angiotensin-converting enzyme inhibitor (ACE) quinapril using the Raij criteria. (a) Arteriolar injury score. (b) Glomerular injury score. (c) Nephrosclerosis score. $^{*}P < 0.0001$ compared with Wistar–Kyoto rats. $^{\dagger}P < 0.0001$ compared with spontaneously hypertensive rats (ANOVA).

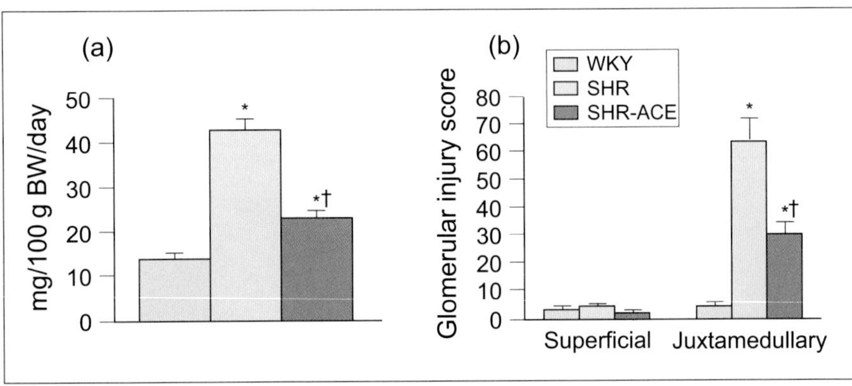

6.11 Relationships between (a) 24-hour urinary protein excretion (UPE) and (b) glomerular injury score (as shown by superficial and juxtaglomerular injury scores) in 73-week-old Wistar–Kyoto rats (WKY) and spontaneously hypertensive rats (SHRs) with naturally developing end-stage renal disease. The SHR were either untreated or were treated with an angiotensin-converting enzyme (ACE) inhibitor for 3 weeks.

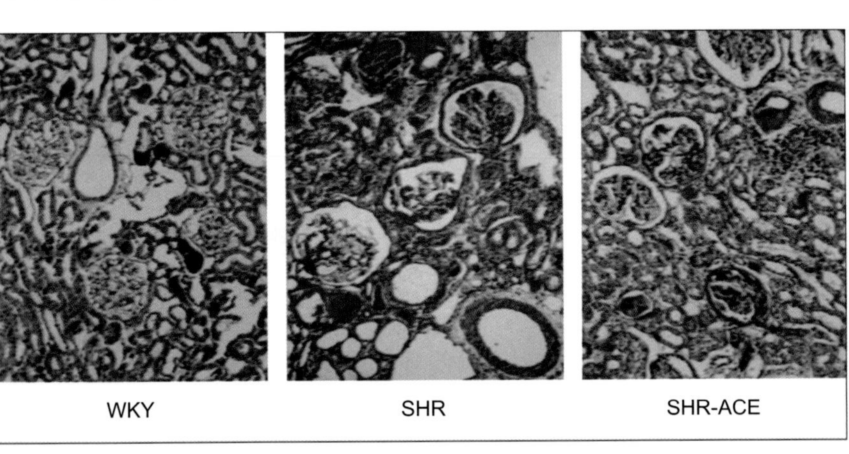

6.12 Representative renal micrographs of 72-week-old normotensive Wistar–Kyoto rats (WKY) and spontaneously hypertensive rats (SHRs) treated for only 3 weeks with an angiotensin-converting enzyme inhibitor.

the disease is exceedingly rapid and severe, the arteriolar lesions present an onion skin appearance that is pathognomonic of malignant nephrosclerosis (**6.13**). As non-malignant hypertensive renal involvement advances, arteriolosclerosis is exacerbated, and the glomeruli exhibit ischaemic wrinkling of the glomerular tuft, thickening of Bowman's capsule, periglomerular fibrosis and glomerular sclerosis; tubular atrophy and interstitial fibrosis also occur.

These pathophysiological changes have been studied in our laboratory under tightly controlled conditions before and after a 3-week course of antihypertensive therapy using the meticulous single-nephron micropuncture techniques described above in various experimental models of hypertension. We found that administration of an ACE inhibitor significantly reduced the arterial and glomerular injury scores (the sum of these two injury indices represents a nephrosclerosis score) (**6.10**) accompanied by a remarkable decrease in urinary protein excretion (**6.11**) and, of course, by physiological renal haemodynamic and glomerular dynamic changes (**6.5** and **6.6**).

One major disadvantage of the above experimental studies is the need to allow SHRs to age for almost 2 years, a very costly and time-consuming practice. As one factor that is common to SHRs and clinical hypertension, ageing, atherosclerosis and nephrosclerosis (**6.14**) is the development of endothelial dysfunction, we repeated the above studies in much younger, 17-week-old, SHRs, but this time adding the nitric oxide synthetase enzyme inhibitor L-NAME (nitro-L-arginine methyl ester hydrochloride) to the drinking water for 3 weeks. Thus, SHRs received tap water only (control), or tap water containing L-NAME with or without the same ACE inhibitor given to the 73-week-old SHRs (**6.15**). An extremely interesting finding was that

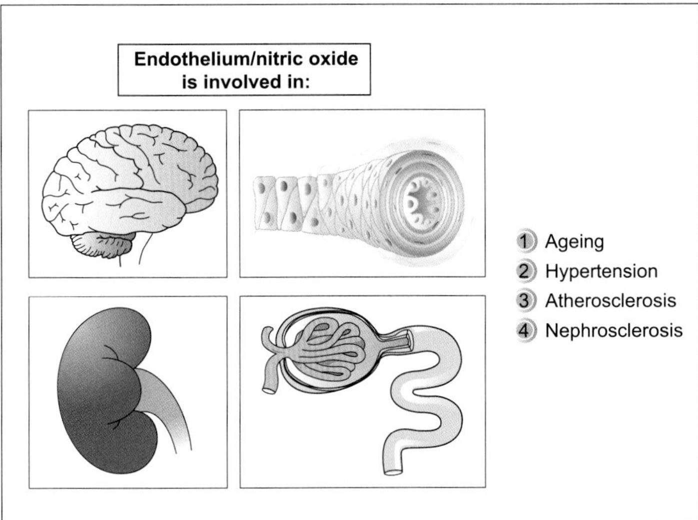

6.14 Endothelial dysfunction of the renal arteries, arterioles and glomerular vessels is common to the nephrosclerosis of hypertension, diabetes, ageing and atherosclerosis.

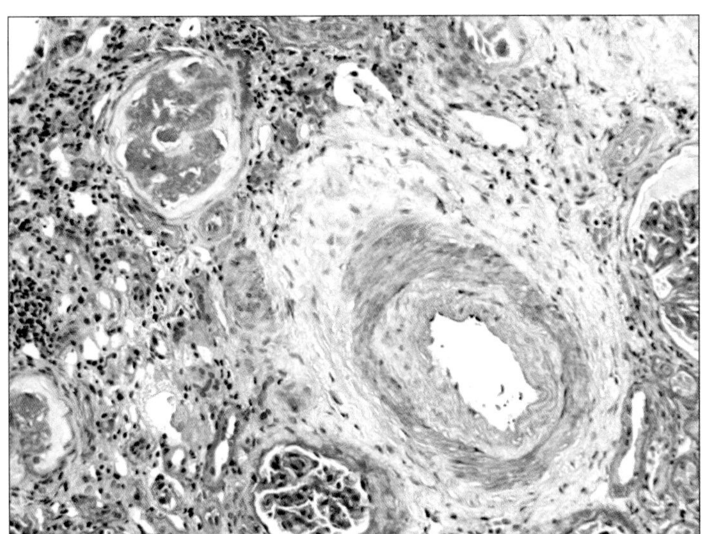

6.13 Large interlobular artery with intimal fibromucoid hyperplasia with perivascular fibrosis. Note irregular thinning of the media. Sclerotic and hyalinized glomeruli with tubular atrophy, irregular fibrosis and chronic inflammation in malignant hypertension are apparent.

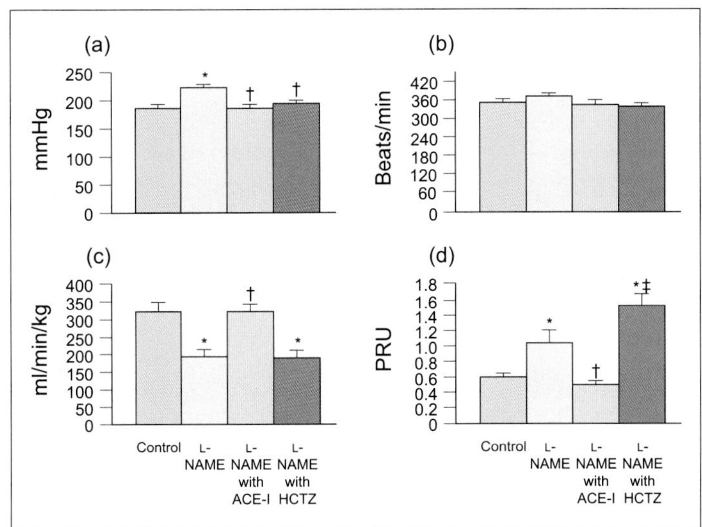

6.15 Systemic haemodynamic changes in control and L-NAME-treated spontaneously hypertensive rats (SHRs) and L-NAME-treated SHRs also administered an ACE inhibitor or hydrochlorothiazide (HCTZ). (a) Mean arterial pressure. (b) Heart rate. (c) Cardiac index. (d) TPRI. *$P < 0.05$ compared with control. †$P < 0.05$ compared with L-NAME. ‡$P \leq 0.01$ compared with angiotensin-converting enzyme inhibitor (ACE-I).

17-week-old SHRs administered L-NAME for only 3 weeks exhibited all of the pathophysiological changes of ESRD that occurred naturally with ageing in 73-week old SHRs (**6.14**–**6.20**).

Thus, when the same ACE inhibitor was co-administered with L-NAME to younger (20-week-old) adult SHRs, the pathophysiological alterations were identical to those observed in the earlier studies of aged (73-week-old) SHRs (**6.15**–**6.20**). The systemic haemodynamic (**6.15**), glomerular dynamics and intrarenal haemodynamics were reversed (**6.16**) pathologically (**6.17**), clinically, (**6.18**), histologically (**6.19**) and immunologically (**6.20**). Of particular note, when another series of younger adult SHRs were treated with a diuretic, hydrochlorothiazide, the dramatic improvements observed in the ACE inhibitor-treated group were not achieved. In fact, further deterioration of renal parenchymal, haemodynamic and dynamic function (**6.15**–**6.20**) that was the complete opposite of the changes observed in animals treated with ACE inhibitor and the diuretic was confirmed pathologically

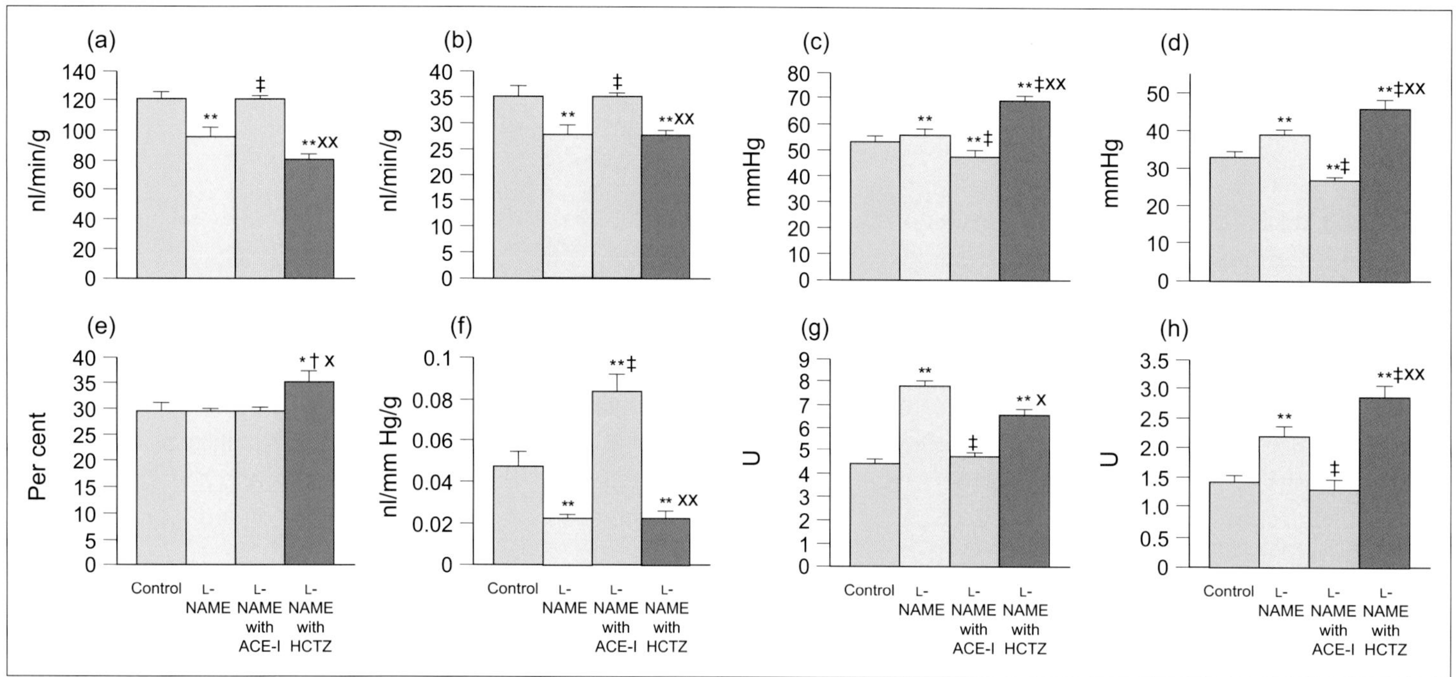

6.16 Glomerular dynamic changes obtained by micropuncture in young adult (20-week-old) spontaneously hypertensive rats (SHRs) given only tap water (control), tap water containing L-NAME or tap water containing L-NAME and either an angiotensin-converting enzyme (ACE) inhibitor or a diuretic (hydrochlorothiazide, HCTZ). (a) Single-nephron plasma flow. (b) Single-nephron glomerular filtration rate. (c) Glomerular hydrostatic pressure. (d) Stopped flow pressure. (e) Single-nephron filtration fraction. (f) Filtration coefficient. (g) Afferent resistance. (h) Efferent resistance. **$P < 0.05$ compared with control. ‡$P < 0.01$ compared with L-NAME. ¥$P < 0.05$, ¥¥$P < 0.01$ compared with ACE-I. *$P < 0.05$, **$P < 0.01$ compared with control. †$P < 0.05$, ‡$P < 0.01$, compared with L-NAME.

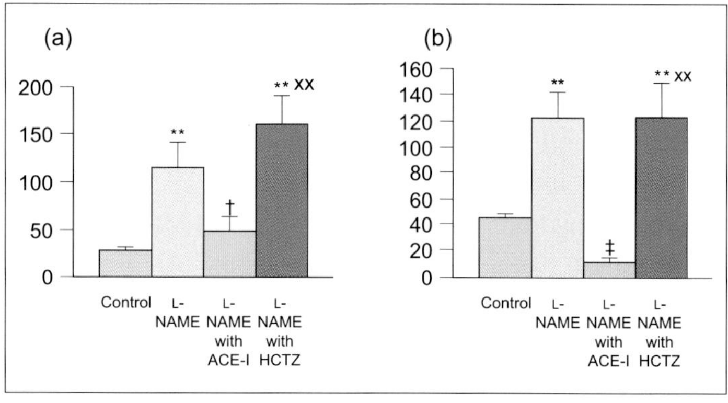

6.17 Pathological changes (glomerular and arteriolar injury scores) obtained in 20-week-old adult spontaneously hypertensive rats administered tap water only (controls), tap water containing L-NAME or tap water containing L-NAME and either an angiotensin-converting enzyme inhibitor (ACE-I) or hydrochlorothiazide (HCTZ). (a) Glomerular injury score. (b) Arteriolar injury score. **$P < 0.01$ vs. control. †$P < 0.05$, ‡$P < 0.01$, compared L-NAME. ¥¥$P < 0.01$ compared with ACE-I.

(**6.17**). Furthermore, in a very recent study, the adverse pathophysiological changes produced by the diuretic were totally prevented by the addition of an ACE inhibitor or an angiotensin II (type 1) receptor blocking agent or both.

These findings strongly suggest that angiotensin II has an important role in the complex mechanisms underlying ESRD and that its inhibition participates favourably in their reversal. Moreover, since the diuretic exacerbated the

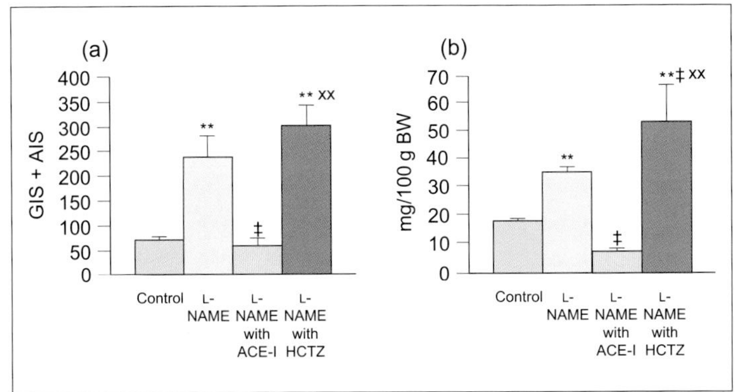

6.18 Relationship between nephrosclerosis score (arteriolar plus glomerular injury scores) and 24-hour urinary protein excretion in 20-week-old spontaneously hypertensive rats given only tap water (controls), tap water containing L-NAME alone or tap water containing L-NAME and an angiotensin-converting enzyme inhibitor (ACE-I) or hydrochlorothiazide (HCTZ) for 3 weeks. (a) Nephrosclerosis score. (b) Urinary protein excretion. $^{**}P < 0.01$ compared with control. $‡P < 0.01$ compared with L-NAME. ¥¥$P < 0.01$ compared with ACE-I.

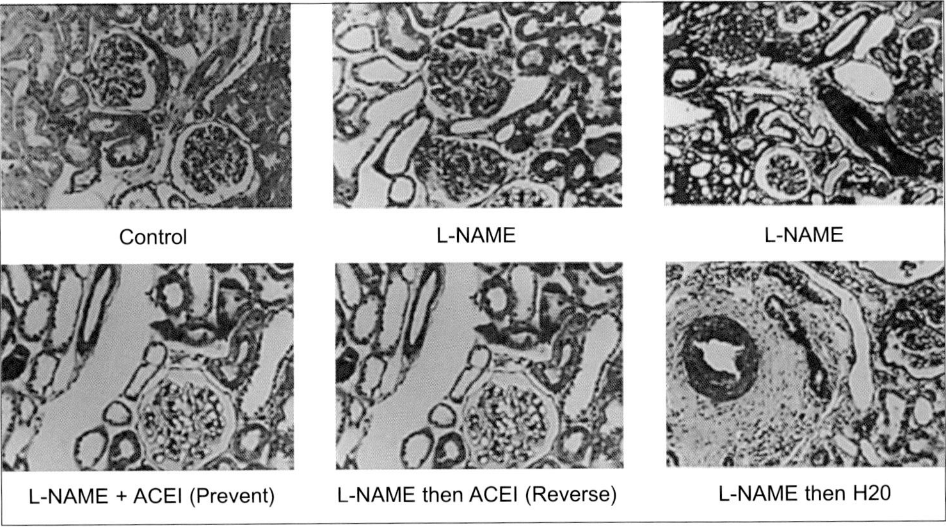

6.19 Histological studies demonstrating the glomerular and arteriolar lesions resulting from administration of L-NAME or L-NAME and an angiotensin-converting enzyme (ACE) inhibitor for 3 weeks. Note the reversal of the lesions with ACE inhibitor but not when tap water was given over 3 weeks after L-NAME had been given for 3 weeks.

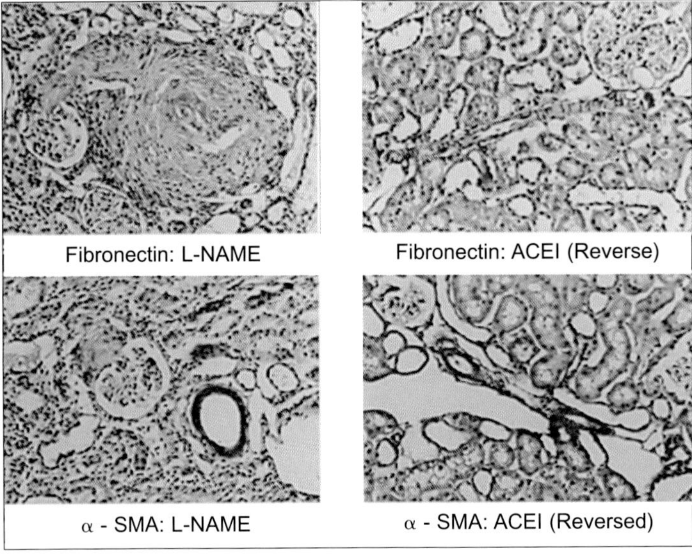

6.20 Immunohistological studies demonstrating the same pathological lesions of the glomeruli and arterioles with L-NAME as occur in clinical nephrosclerosis and their reversal with an ACE inhibitor. Renal tissue was stained for fibronectin or α-smooth muscle actin (SMA).

findings of ESRD, this suggests that it may have stimulated the local renal renin–angiotensin system. This concept was suggested further by our recent findings that demonstrated that these thiazide-induced adverse findings were prevented by co-treatment with an agent(s) that inhibits the renin–angiotensin system.

In yet another study, when HOE-140 (icatibant), a bradykinin receptor antagonist, was co-administered with an ACE inhibitor, the responses were no different from those obtained with the ACE inhibitor alone, suggesting that bradykinin did not play a significant role in the beneficial effects of the ACE inhibitor or, for that matter, an angiotensin II (type 1) receptor (AT_1) antagonist. Finally, since the effects of the ACE inhibitor and the AT_1 receptor antagonist were very similar, we suggest that both agents acted in a similiar fashion on the kidney, by antagonizing the renin–angiotensin system (**6.21**–**6.24**).

In other studies, we observed that blockers of three

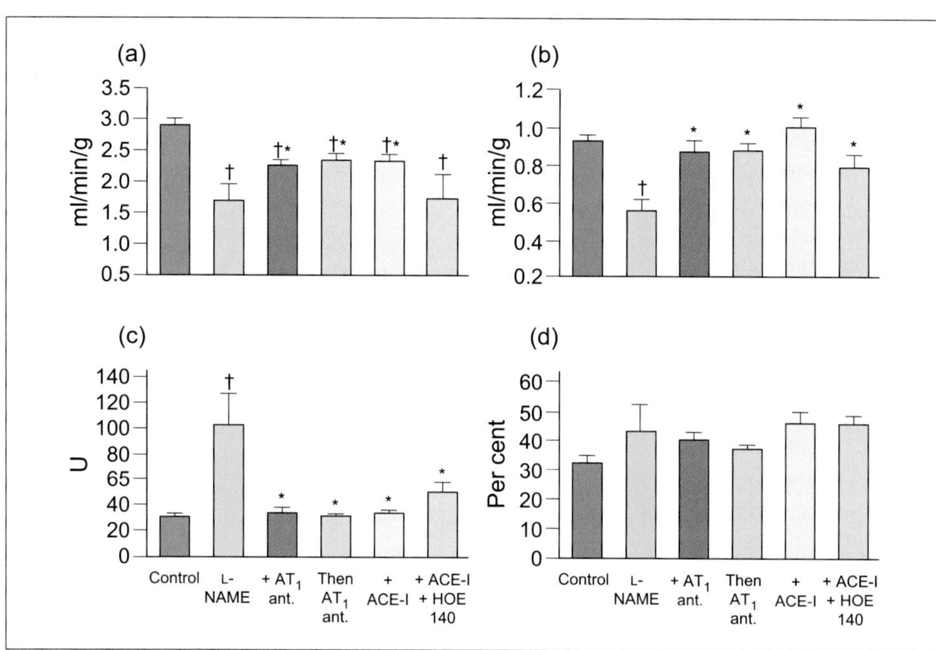

6.21 Whole-kidney haemodynamics in control spontaneously hypertensive rats (receiving tap water alone) and rats treated with L-NAME, L-NAME plus an angiotensin II type 1 (AT_1) receptor antagonist, with L-NAME for 3 weeks and then the AT_1 receptor antagonist, with L-NAME plus an angiotensin-converting enzyme (ACE) inhibitor or with L-NAME plus ACE inhibitor plus HOE-140 (icatibant). (a) Estimated renal plasma flow. (b) Glomerular filtration rate. (c) Renal vascular resistance. (d) Filtration fraction.

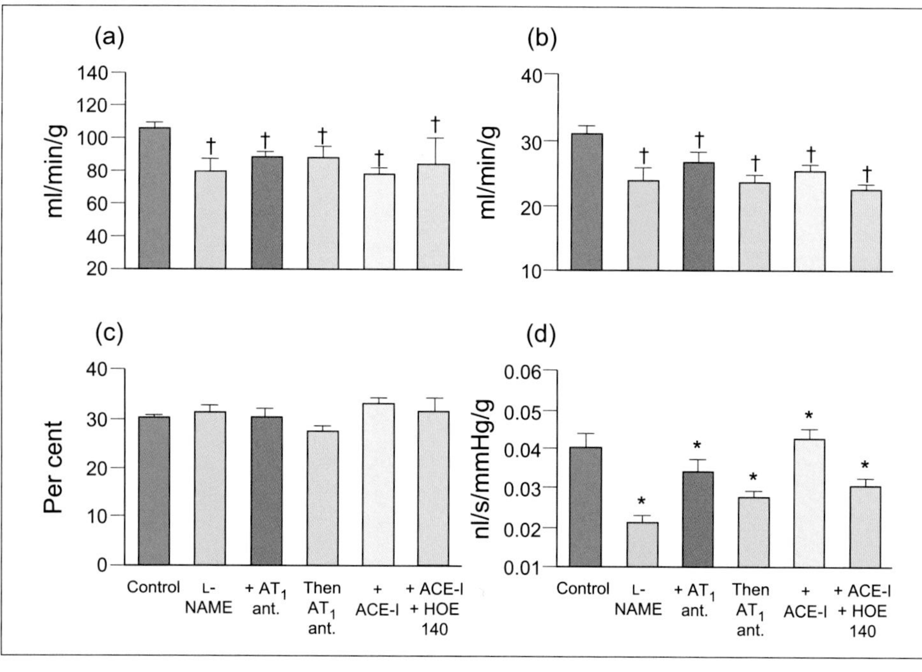

6.22 Glomerular haemodynamics in spontaneously hypertensive rats treated as described in **6.21**. (a) Single-nephron plasma flow. (b) Single-nephron glomerular filtration rate. (c) Single-nephron filtration fraction. (d) Filtration coefficient.

6.23 Glomerular dynamic responses in spontaneously hypertensive rats treated as described in **6.21**. (a) Afferent glomerular arteriolar resistance. (b) Efferent glomerular arteriolar resistance.
(c) Glomerular hydrostatic pressure.
(d) Stopped flow pressure.

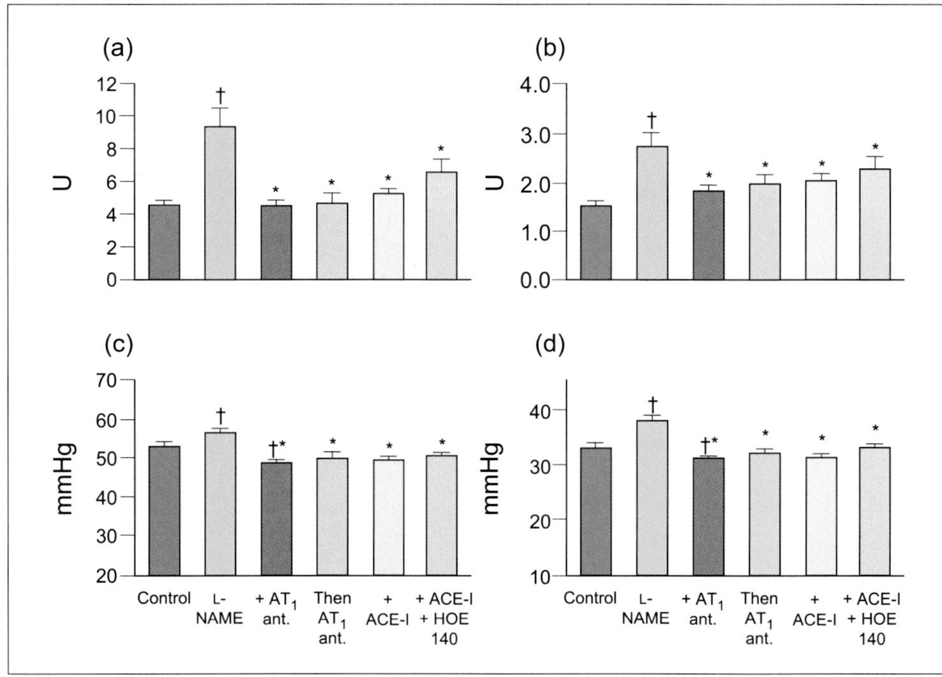

6.24 Renal function and pathophysiology in spontaneously hypertensive rats treated as described in **6.21** (a) Glomerular injury score. (b) Arteriolar injury score. (c) Serum creatinine concentration. (d) Twenty-four-hour urinary protein excretion.

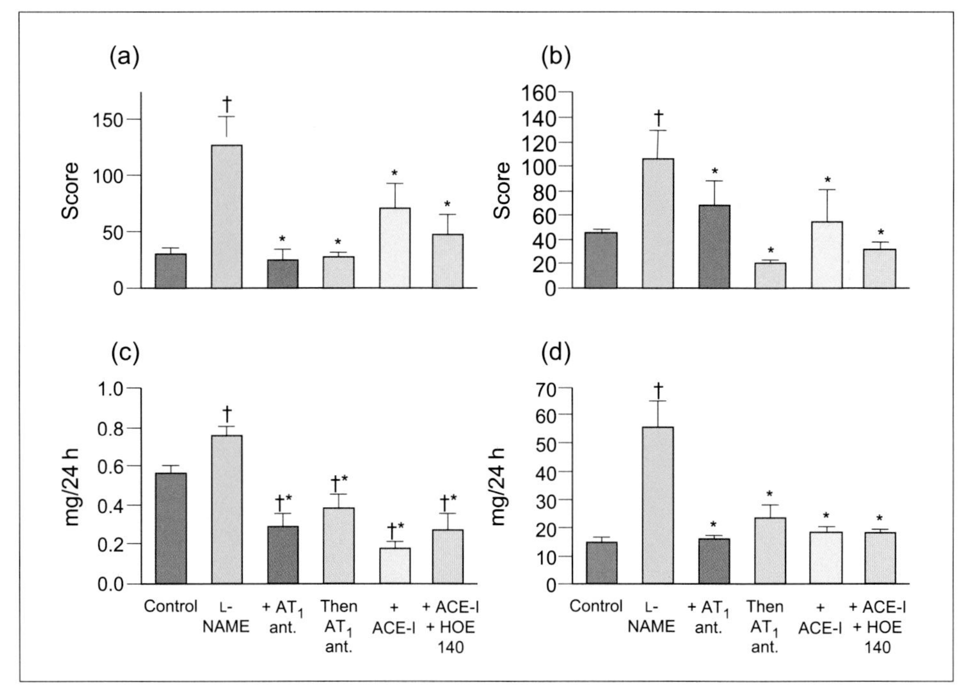

different types of calcium antagonist (an L-, N- or T-type) produced similar findings under the same experimental conditions (**6.25–6.28**).

Finally, to demonstrate further the important role of nitric oxide synthesis on renal vascular and glomerular function, we administered the essential amino acid precursor, L-arginine, required for nitric oxide synthesis. The L-arginine was administered to 85-week-old SHRs for 3 weeks and, although extensive renal micropuncture studies could not be performed in these very old rats, it was possible to measure systemic and whole-kidney haemodynamics (**6.28**). Furthermore, treatment with L-arginine

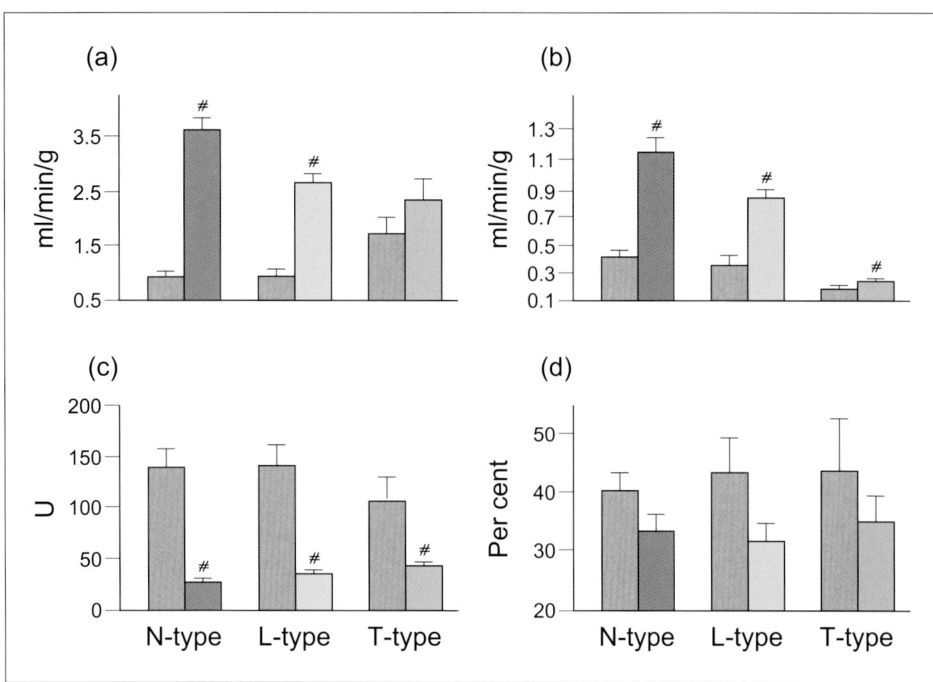

6.25 Comparison of the effects of three types of calcium antagonists (N-, L- and T-type) on whole-kidney haemodynamics in 17-week-old spontaneously hypertensive rats (SHRs) co-treated with L-NAME for 3 weeks. Open bars: control SHRs given only tap water; shaded bars: SHRs treated with each type of calcium channel antagonist. (a) Estimated renal plasma flow. (b) Glomerular filtration rate. (c) Renal vascular resistance. (d) Filtration fraction.

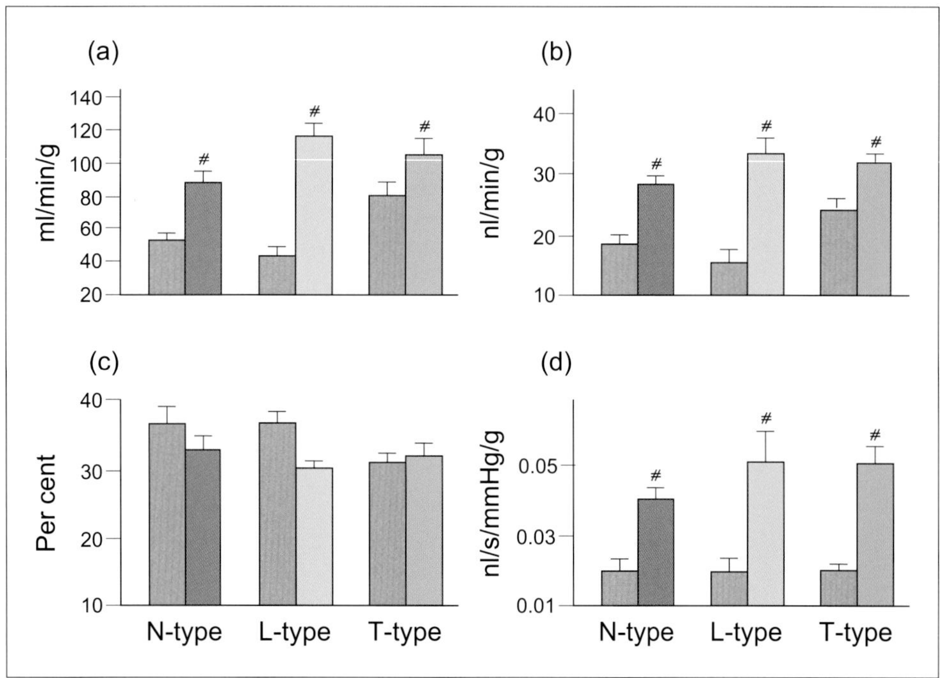

6.26 Comparison of the effects of three types of calcium antagonists (N-, L- and T-type) on glomerular dynamics in 17-week-old spontaneously hypertensive rats (SHRs) co-treated with L-NAME for 3 weeks. Open bars: control SHRs given only tap water; shaded bars: SHRs treated with each type of calcium antagonist. (a) Single-nephron plasma flow. (b) Single-nephron glomerular filtration rate. (c) Single-nephron filtration fraction. (d) Filtration fraction.

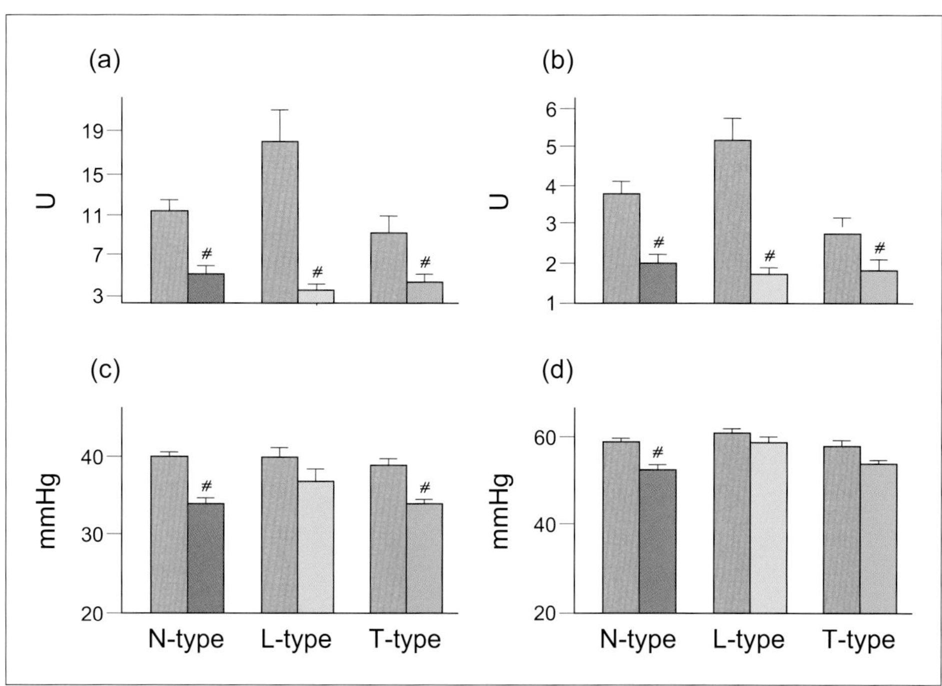

6.27 Comparison of the effects three types of calcium antagonists (N-, L- and T-type) on glomerular dynamics) in 17-week-old spontaneously hypertensive rats (SHRs) co-treated with L-NAME for 3 weeks. Open bars: SHRs given only tap water; shaded bars: SHRs treated with each type of calcium antagonist. (a) Afferent glomerular arteriolar resistance. (b) Efferent glomerular arteriolar resistance. (c) Stopped flow pressure. (d) Glomerular hydrostatic pressure.

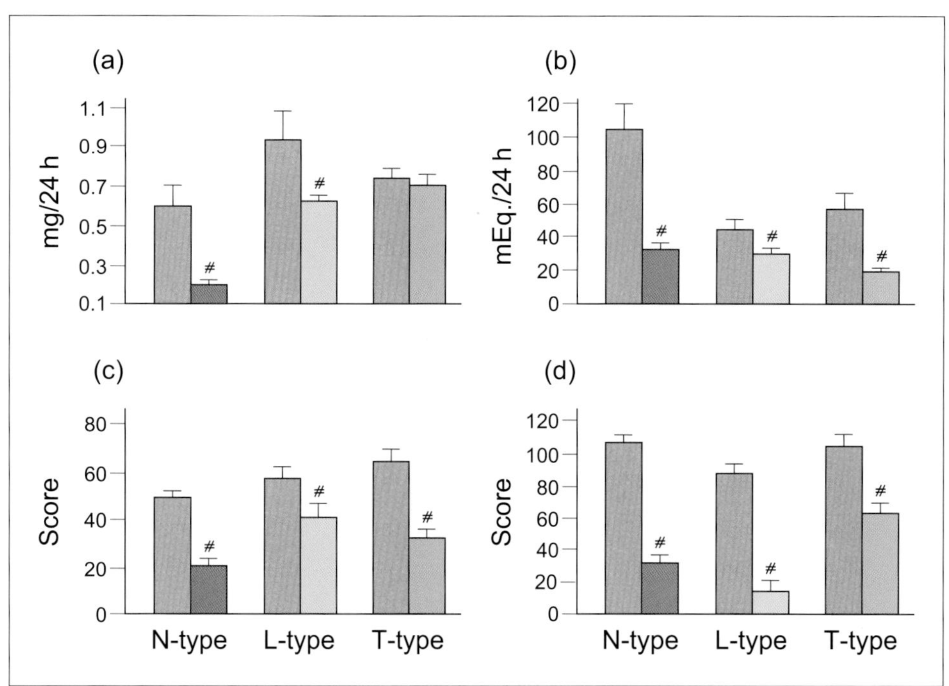

6.28 Comparison of the effects of three types of calcium antagonists (N-, L- and T-type) on hepatic function and pathology in 17-week-old spontaneously hypertensive rats (SHRs) co-treated with L-NAME for 3 weeks. Open bars: SHRs given only tap water; shaded bars: SHRs treated with each type of calcium antagonist. (a) Serum creatinine concentration. (b) Twenty-four-hour urinary protein excretion. (c) Glomerular injury index. (d) Arteriolar injury index.

also reduced the severity of the arteriolar disease and glomerular injury scoring and resulted in a decreased 24-hour urinary protein excretion and rises in the serum creatinine and uric acid concentration (*Tables 6.3* and *6.4* and **6.29** and **6.30**).

The renal functional and histological studies described above demonstrate that the renal lesions that occur in naturally occurring SHRs, either spontaneously or as a result of the inhibition of nitric oxide synthesis, were preventable, were not primarily pressure dependent and may be treatable with specific drugs. In addition, the findings strongly suggest that ESRD can be explained (at least in part) by renal vascular and glomerular endothelial dysfunction arising from a defect in nitric oxide synthesis.

The clinical relevance of this series of experiments has been substantiated by a number of reports from several multicentre clinical trials that have confirmed that a variety of ACE inhibitors and AT_1 antagonists have similar pathophysiological efficacy. Thus, first ACE inhibitors (**6.31** and **6.32**)

Table 6.3 Systemic and renal haemodynamics before and after L-arginine in 85-week-old spontaneously hypertensive rats

Index	*SHR*	*SHR + L-Arginine*
MAP (mmHg)	188 ± 14	173 ± 9
CI (ml/min/kg)	187 ± 26	263 ± 15*
Total peripheral resistance index (U)	1.15 ± 0.18	0.67± 0.06*
ERPF (ml/min)	1.25 ± 0.26	2.03 ± 0.35*
GFR (ml/min)	0.4 ± 0.07	0.79 ± 0.07*
FF (%)	36 ± 4	42 ± 4*

*$P < 0.05$, at least.

Table 6.4 Glomerular, arteriolar and nephrosclerosis scores, proteinuria and renal function in 85-week-old untreated and L-arginine-treated spontaneously hypertensive rats

Index	*SHR*	*SHR + L-Arginine*	*P <*
Glomerular injury score			
Subcapsular	50 ± 7	14 ± 4*	0.0005
Juxtamedullary	114 ± 17	69 ± 7	0.05
Total	164 ± 22	83 ± 9	0.005
Arteriolar	106 ± 17	102 ± 10	NS
Urinary protein excretion (mg/100 g body weight/24 h)	39 ± 5	19 ± 5	0.05
Serum creatinine (mg/dl)	1.4 ± 0.1	0.9 ± 0.1	0.05
Serum uric acid (mg/dl)	1.8 ± 0.4	1.8 ± 0.4	NS

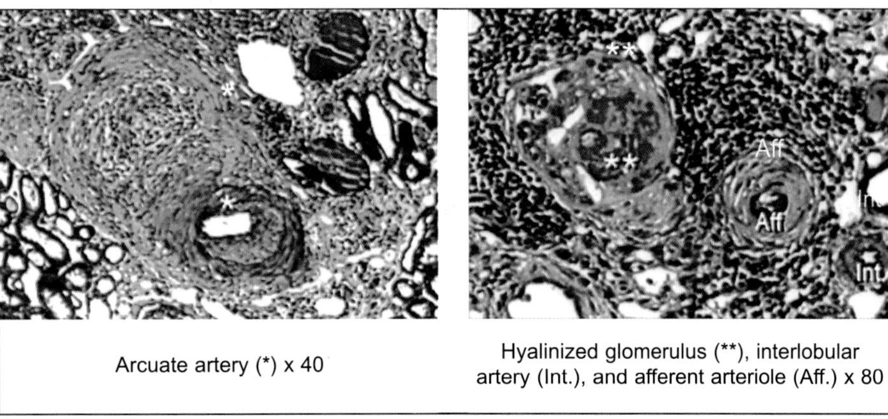

Arcuate artery (*) x 40

Hyalinized glomerulus (**), interlobular artery (Int.), and afferent arteriole (Aff.) x 80

6.29 Demonstration of the severe hypertensive nephrosclerosis in 85-week old spontaneously hypertensive rats. Presented on the left is the severe malignant accurate artery disease; on the right are an hyalinized glomerulus, interlobular artery (Int) and afferent arteriole (Aff).

6.30 The effect of 3 weeks' L-arginine administration on the renal pathology of 85-week old spontaneously hypertensive rats (SHRs). Left: effects of severe (malignant) nephrosclerosis in untreated SHRs; right: effects of L-arginine treatment in drinking water (3 weeks). Note the prevention of glomerular and tubular injury.

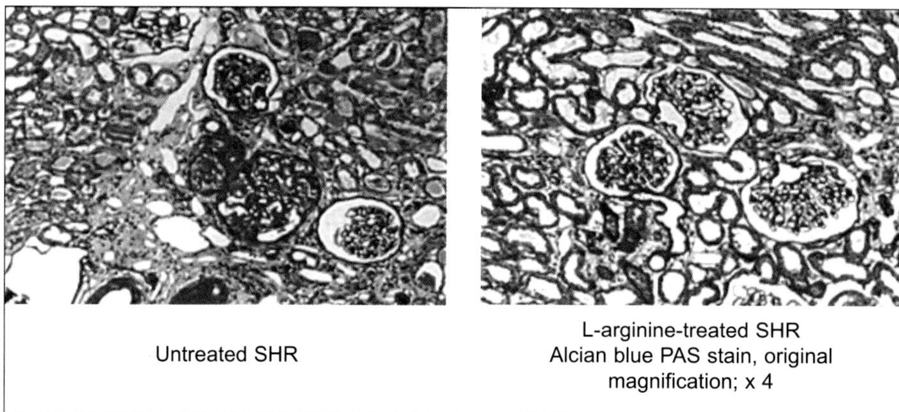

6.31 Effects of placebo or captopril on the cumulative incidence of renal events in patients with diabetes. Note the significant reduction in (a) the percentage of patients in whom baseline creatinine concentration was doubled and (b) the number of patients who died or required dialysis or renal transplantation. This is the first trial demonstrating the effectiveness of an angiotensin-converting enzyme inhibitor in reducing indicators of end-stage renal disease. Reproduced with permission from Lewis EJ, Hunsickeer LG, Bain RP, Rhode RD: The effect of angiotensin-converting-enzyme inhibition on diabetic nephropathy. The Collaborative Study Group. *N. Engl. J. Med.* 1993;**320**:1456–1462.

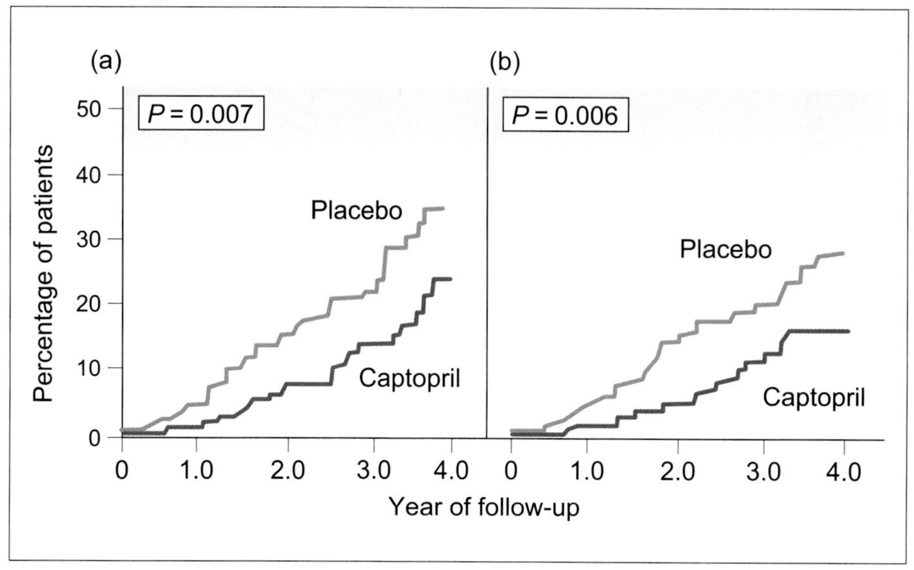

6.32 Results of a second angiotensin-converting enzyme (ACE) inhibitor trial (HOPE study) comparing the effects of ramipril and placebo on (a) myocardial infarction, stroke and death from cardiovascular causes and (b) albuminuria in hypertensive and/or diabetic patients.

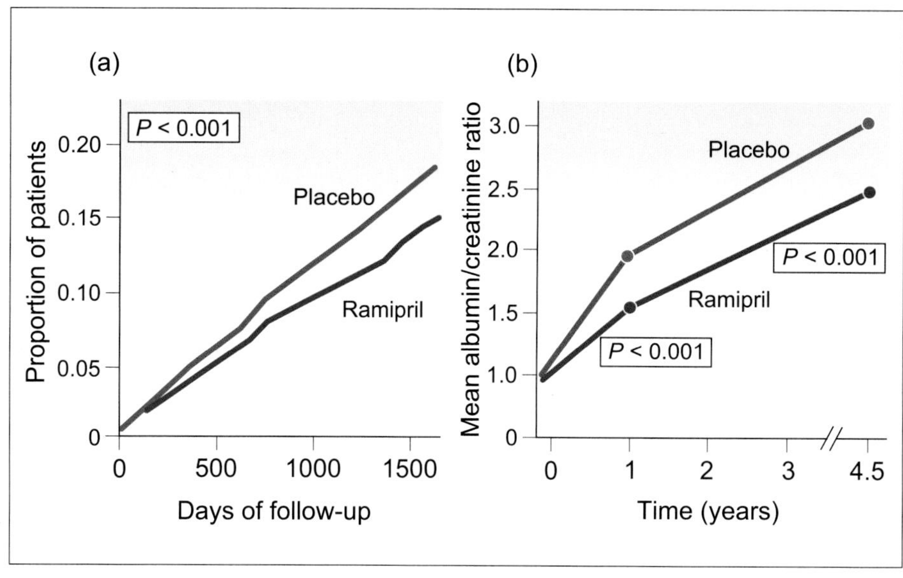

and then AT_1 antagonists (**6.33**–**6.35**) have been found to slow significantly the progression of renal functional impairment, urinary protein excretion and, eventually, ESRD.

The first ACE inhibitor and AT_1 antagonist studies demonstrating efficacy in patients with ESRD were conducted in patients with hypertension and diabetes or cardiac failure. However, an excellent meta-analysis of clinical studies has clearly demonstrated that ACE inhibitors are indicated for the treatment of non-diabetic patients with chronic renal disease and proteinuria (*Box 6.1*).

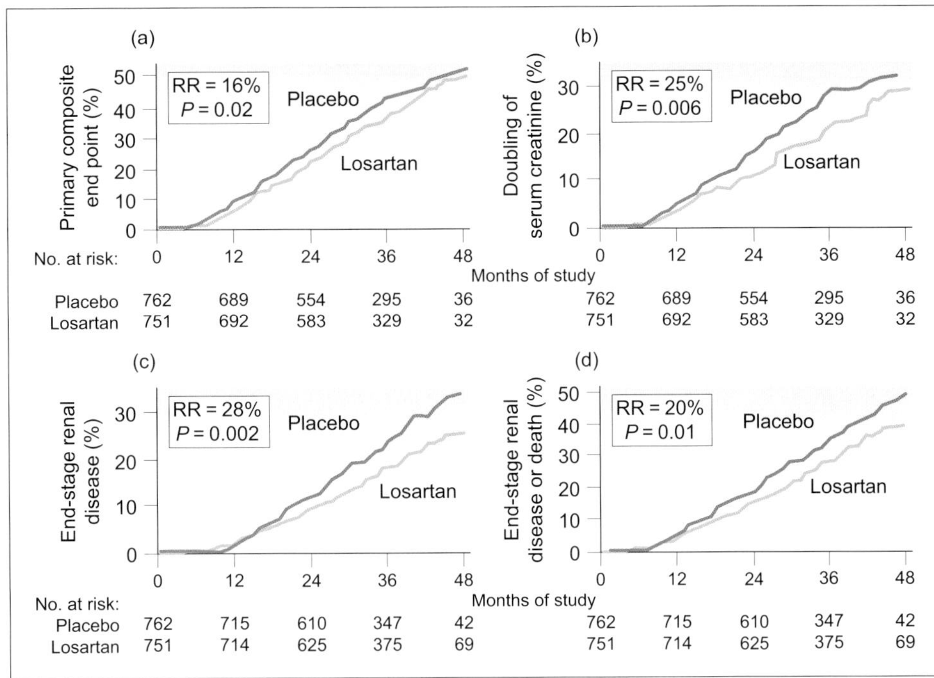

6.33 Effects of the angiotensin II type receptor 1 (AT_1) antagonist losartan on renal and cardiovascular outcomes in patients with type 2 diabetes. Reproduced with permission from Brenner BM, Cooper ME, de Zeeuw D, Keane WF, Parving HH, *et al.*: Effects of losartan on renal and cardiovascular outcomes in patients with type 2 diabetes and nephropathy. *N. Engl. J. Med.* 2001;**345**:861–869.

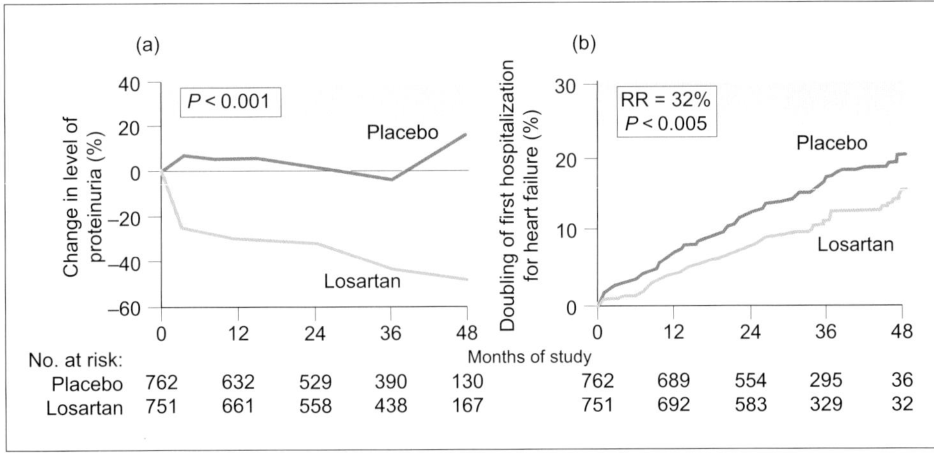

6.34 Effects of the angiotensin II type receptor 1 (AT_1) antagonist losartan on (a) median change from baseline in the level of proteinuria and (b) percentage of patients with a first hospitalization for heart failure. Reproduced with permission from Brenner BM *et al.* (as above).

Box 6.1 Angiotensin-converting enzyme inhibitors and progression of non-diabetic disease

'Conclusion: Antihypertensive regiment that include ACE inhibitors are more effective than regimens without ACE inhibitors in slowing the progression of nondiabetic renal disease. The beneficial effect of ACE inhibitors is mediated by factors in addition to decreasing blood pressure and urinary protein excretion and is greater in patients with proteinuria. Angiotensin-converting inhibitors are indicated for treatment of nondiabetic patients with chronic renal disease and proteinuria and, possibly, those without proteinuria.'

Tazeen *et al.* (2001)

Not all of the molecular/cellular mechanisms involved in the prevention and reversal of renal involvement in hypertension or diabetes with the agents above described are clearly known. However, they must be exceedingly complex and primarily involve inhibition of the renin–angiotensin system, cytokines, growth factors and other pathways. Thus far, it seems plain that activation of the intrarenal renin–angiotensin system contributes to the development and progression of nephrosclerosis. Clearly, then, angiotensin II is a major factor that promotes the pathological changes of arteriolar nephrosclerosis through haemodynamic as well as non-haemodynamic mechanisms that involve progressive vasoconstriction and mitogenic and profibrogenetic actions that result in the production of extracellular matrix component, inflammatory responses and other responses linked to fibrogenic cytokines (e.g. transforming growth factor β). Additionally, reduced nitric oxide availability obviously occurs due to downregulation of endothelial nitric oxide synthesis activity and increased oxidative stress. To our way of thinking, these therapeutic changes are not solely based on reduction in arterial pressure to lower goal blood pressure levels, although several multicentre trials attest to the importance of exquisite control of arterial pressure. Recently, we demonstrated that when the aldosterone receptor blocking agent eplerenone was administered along with L-NAME, no significant haemodynamic responses were obtained although glomerular and arteriolar injury scores were

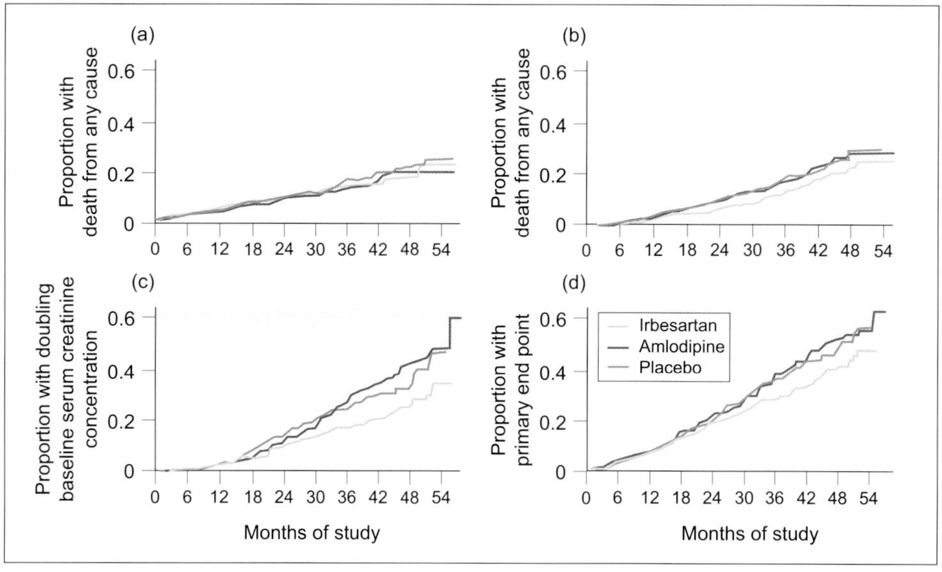

6.35 Effects of another angiotensin receptor blocker on renal function in patients with type 2 diabetes mellitus. (a) Death from any cause. (b) End-stage renal disease. (c) Doubling of baseline serum creatinine concentration. (d) Primary composite end point. Reproduced with permission form Lewis *et al.* (1993).

profoundly improved, as was tubular interstitial damage (**6.36–6.41**).

Thus, haemodynamic factors and the expression of angiotensin II actions do not constitute the 'final story'; other factors will no doubt prove to be incredibly important as the story unfolds.

Role of uric acid

In recent years, interest in the role of uric acid in the pathogenesis of essential hypertension has undergone a resurgence. There are those who feel that this metabolic product is a pathogenetic factor in the development of renal

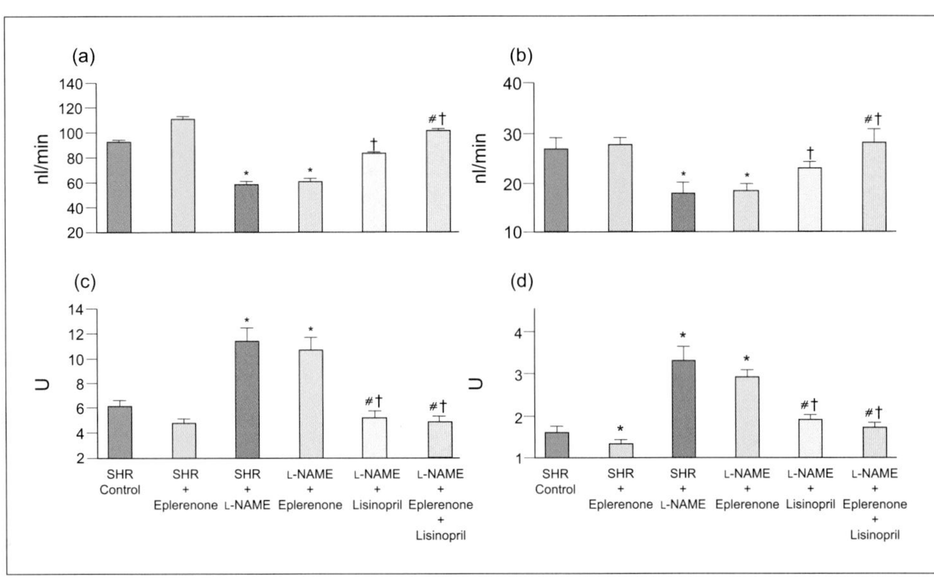

6.36 Glomerular dynamic changes in control spontaneously hypertensive rats (SHRs) and those produced by eplerenone, L-NAME, L -NAME plus eplerenone, L-NAME plug lisinopril and L-NAME plus lisinopril and eplerenone. (a) Single-nephron plasma flow. (b) Single-nephron glomerular filtration rate. (c) Afferent renal resistance. (d) Efferent renal resistance. $^*P < 0.05$ compared with SHR controls. $†P < 0.05$ compared with L-NAME/SHR. $\#P < 0.05$ compared with L-NAME/SHR plus eplerenone.

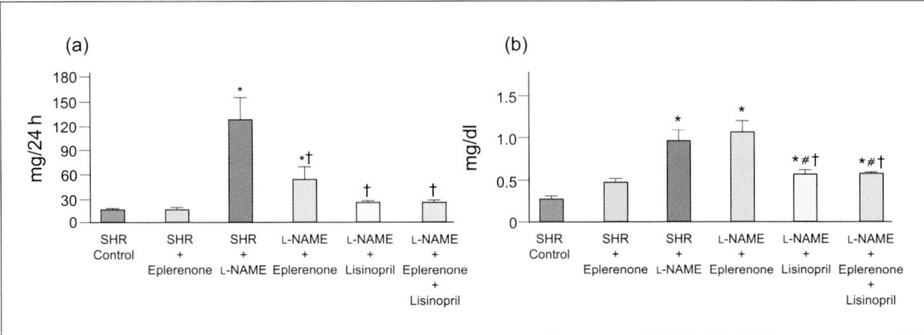

6.37 (a) Twenty-four-hour urinary protein excretion and (b) serum creatinine concentration in control spontaneously hypertensive rats (SHRs) and those treated with eplerenone, L-NAME, L-NAME plus eplerenone, L-NAME plus lisinopril or L-NAME plus lisinopril and eplerenone. $^*P < 0.05$ compared with SHR control. $†P < 0.05$ compared with L-NAME/SHR. $\#P < 0.05$ compared with L-NAME/SHR plus eplerenone.

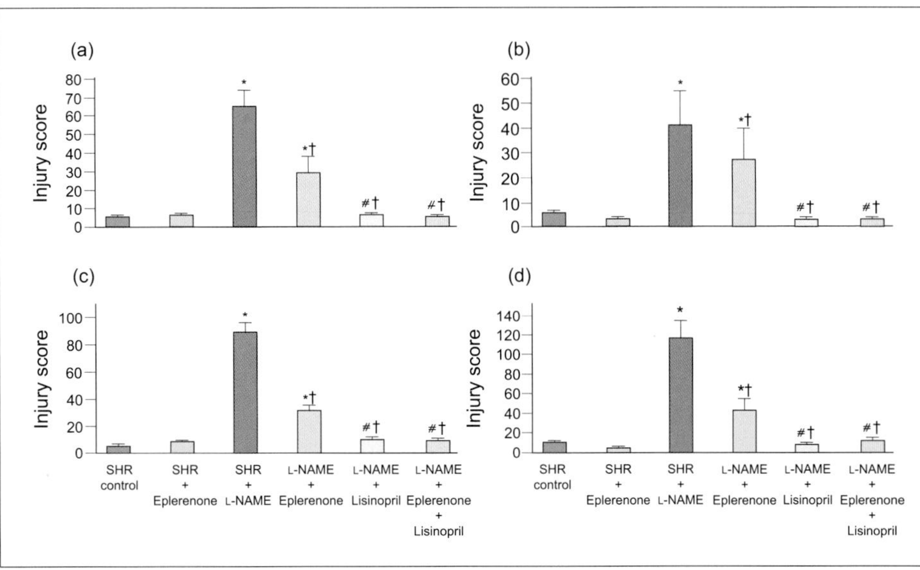

6.38 Renal histopathological changes in control rats and rats treated with L-NAME or eplerenone or L-NAME plus eplerenone, lisinopril or lisinopril and eplerenone. (a) Total glomerular injury score. (b) Subcapsular glomerular injury score (c) Juxtaglomerular injury score. (d) Arteriolar injury score. $^*P < 0.05$ vs. SHR control. $†P < 0.05$ compared with L-NAME/SHR. $\#P < 0.05$ compared with L-NAME/SHR plus eplerenone.

involvement, whereas others believe that the increased serum uric acid concentration observed in patients hypertension is an excellent biomarker of the progression of renal vascular involvement. Indeed, many years ago, before the advent of diuretic therapy, investigators demonstrated the high prevalence of hyperuricaemia in patients with essential hypertension. We have been involved with this issue for many years and have demonstrated, in a large number of patients with uncomplicated essential hypertension, normal renal function and no ECG evidence of left ventricular hypertrophy (LVH), that peak serum uric acid concentration is inversely related to renal blood flow and directly related to the increase in renal vascular resistance (**6.42**). Moreover, in another study, in patients

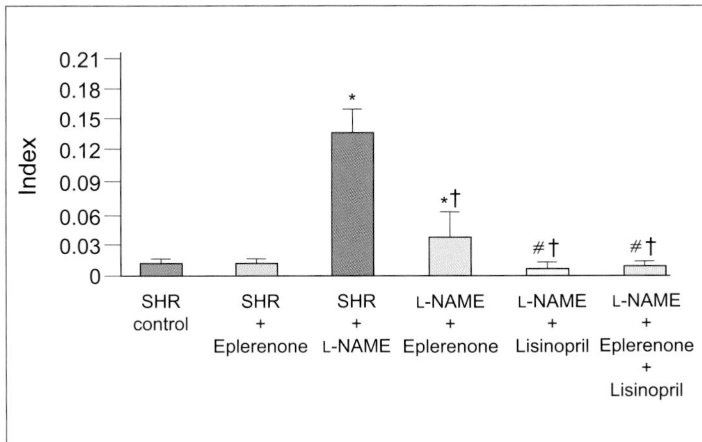

6.39 Tubulointerstitial damage indices observed in control spontaneously hypertensive rats (SHRs) and SHRs treated with eplerenone, L -NAME, L -NAME plus eplerinone, L -NAME plus lisinopril or L -NAME plus lisinopril plus eplerinone. *P < 0.05 compared with SHR control. †P < 0.05 compared with L-NAME/SHR. #P < 0.05 compared with L-NAME/SHR plus eplerenone.

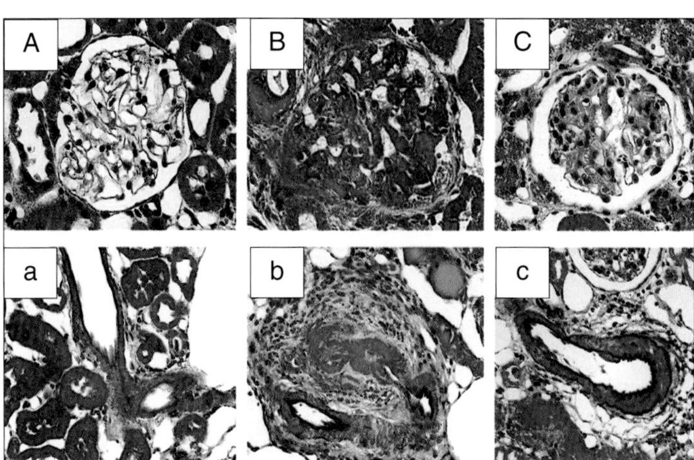

6.40 Glomerular (A–C) and arteriolar (a–c) histological changes observed in (A, a) control spontaneously hypertensive rats, (B, b) spontaneously hypertensive rats treated with L-NAME (and (C, c) spontaneously hypertensive rats treated with the aldosterone antagonist eplerenone.

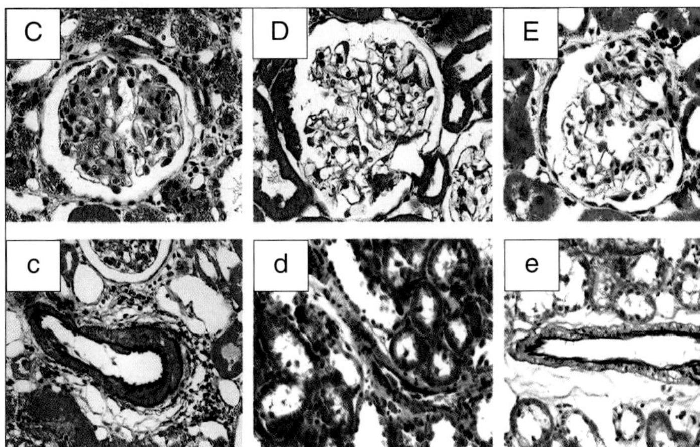

6.41 Molecular (C–E) and arteriolar (c–e) histological changes in spontaneously hypertensive rats treated with L -NAME for 3 weeks in addition to (C, c) the aldosterone antagonist eplerenone, (D, d) the ACE inhibitor lisinopril or (E, e) both. The damage was prevented independent of any beneficial haemodynamic or glomerular dynamic changes.

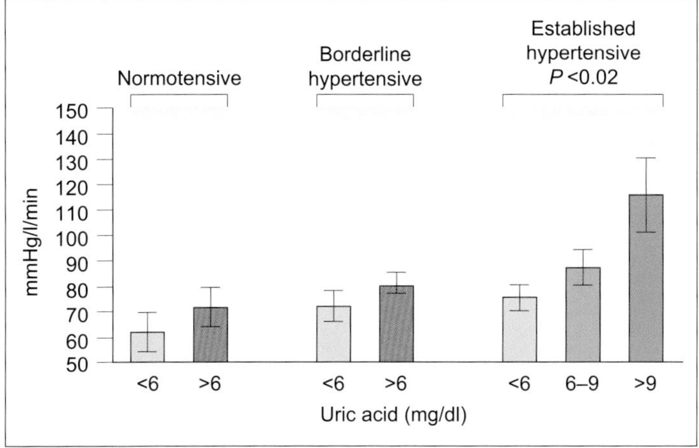

6.42 The direct relationship between serum uric acid concentration and renal vascular resistance in patients with uncomplicated essential hypertension. The relationship in normotensive subjects and in patients with borderline hypertension is also presented.

with echocardiographic evidence of LVH (but with a normal ECG), we found that distribution of cardiac output to the kidney, renal blood flow and uric acid concentration was normal (**6.43**). However, in patients in whom there was clear-cut haemodynamic evidence of a reduced distribution of cardiac output to the kidney, there was definite echocardiographic evidence of LVH (**6.44**) and uric acid levels were significantly higher than in patients in whom distribution of cardiac output to the kidneys was normal (**6.44** and **6.45**).

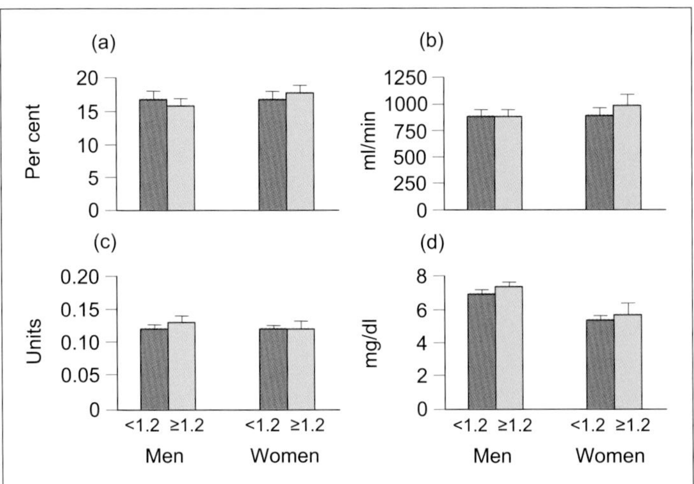

6.43 Renal haemodynamic characteristics of patients with (pulmonary wall thickness [PWT] ≥ 1.2 cm) or without (PWT < 1.2 cm) left ventricular hypertension. (a) Renal distribution of cardiac output. (b) Renal blood flow. (c) Renal vascular resistance. (d) Serum uric acid.

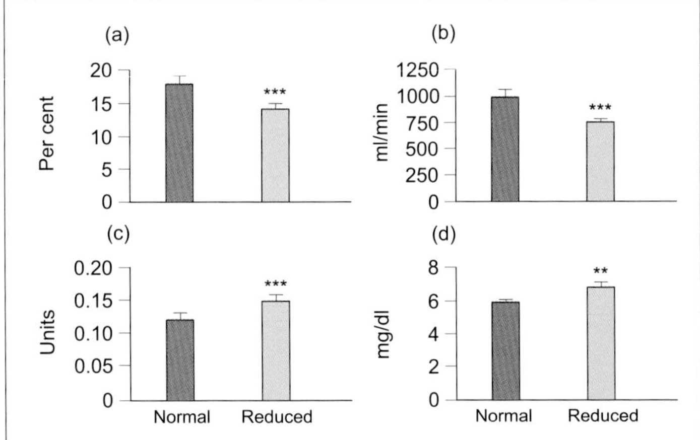

6.44 Renal haemodynamic characteristics of patients with normal (> 16%) or reduced (≤ 16%) renal blood flow/cardiac output ratio. (a) Renal distribution of cardiac output. (b) Renal blood flow. (c) Renal vascular resistance. (d) Serum uric acid. ***P* < 0.02. ****P* < 0.01.

Furthermore, in patients with elevated serum uric acid levels, distribution of cardiac output to the kidney was reduced and LVH was apparent on echocardiography (**6.45**). These findings provide exceedingly strong evidence that cardiac involvement in hypertension precedes renal haemodynamic involvement. In fact, these findings are not consistent with the general statements that microalbuminuria (or proteinuria) precedes or predicts cardiovascular involvement in hypertension or, for that matter, coronary heart disease. It should be recognized that the increase in protein excretion that occurs in patients with renal involvement is actually evidence of vascular involvement of the kidney.

We concluded from these findings that the serum uric acid concentration is an excellent clinical index of early-developing nephrosclerosis (in the absence of those other factors that may produce hyperuricaemia). Furthermore, when we studied other patients with occlusive renal arterial disease and hypertension, and subsequently corrected their renal arterial lesions, we found that the uric acid level decreased following the repair of the lesion.

These data are further supported by many epidemiological reports involving patients with coronary heart disease. As a group, these patients had higher serum uric acid concentration, which was an excellent index (a minor risk factor, if you will) of the severity of the CHD. We have interpreted these findings to represent the presence of systemic vascular disease with increased arteriolar resistance.

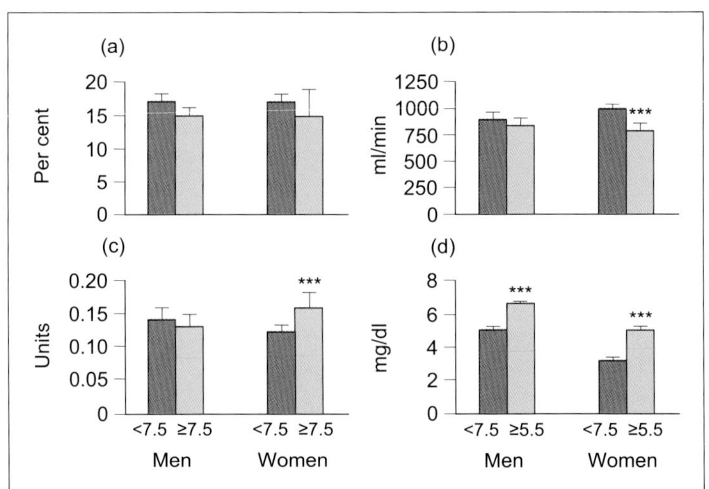

6.45 Renal haemodynamics of patients with or without increased serum uric acid level. (a) Renal distribution of cardiac output. (b) Renal blood flow. (c) Renal vascular resistance. (d) Serum uric acid. **P* < 0.05. ****P* < 0.01.

Supporting this line of thinking, a number of years ago investigators infused either norepinephrine or angiotensin II into normotensive subjects. The ensuing rise in arterial pressure during these infusions was accompanied by an increase in serum uric acid concentration, associated with diminished renal blood flow and glomerular filtration rate. Then, when the infusion was discontinued and arterial pressure returned to normal pretreatment levels, the uric acid concentrations also normalized, as did their renal blood flows and glomerular filtration rates. Thus, our purpose in including this information in this chapter is to present an alternative argument to the currently advanced concept that elevated uric acid levels in patients with essential hypertension are a pathogenetic index of intrarenal vascular involvement from hypertensive disease. Moreover, we strongly believe that the serum uric acid level is an excellent clinical marker of the state of intrarenal arteriolar constriction or the height of arterial pressure; and we have found this to be a most useful index in the long-term follow-up of our patients with hypertension.

Further reading

Papers related to illustrations

Uchino, K, Frohlich, ED, Nishikimi, T, Isshiki, T, Kardon, MB: Spontaneously hypertensive rats demonstrate increased renal vascular alpha-$_1$ adrenergic receptor responsiveness. *Am. J. Physiol.* 1991;**260**:R889–R893. *This paper involves the use of the Gomez formulae for determining renal and glomerular dynamics.*

Komatsu K, Frohlich ED, Ono H, Ono Y, Numabe A, Willis GW: Glomerular dynamics and morphology of aged SHR: Effects of angiotensin converting enzyme inhibitor. *Hypertension* 1995;**25**:207–213.

Ono H, Ono Y, Frohlich ED: Nitric oxide synthase inhibition in spontaneously hypertensive rats: systemic, renal, and glomerular hemodynamics. *Hypertension* 1995;**26**:249–255.

Ono H, Ono Y, Frohlich ED: ACE inhibition prevents and reverses L-NAME exacerbated nephrosclerosis in spontaneously hypertensive rats. *Hypertension* 1996;**27**:176–183.

Ono Y, Ono H, Frohlich ED: Hydrochlorothiazide exacerbates nitric oxide-blockade nephrosclerosis with glomerular hypertension in spontaneously hypertensive rats. *J. Hypertens.* 1996;**14**:823–828.

Ono H, Ono Y, Frohlich ED: L-Arginine reverses severe nephrosclerosis in aged spontaneously hypertensive rats. *J. Hypertens.* 1999;**17**:121–128.

Nakamura Y, Ono H, Frohlich ED: Differential effects of T- and L-type calcium antagonists on glomerular dynamics in spontaneously hypertensive rats. *Hypertension* 1999;**34**:273–278.

Nakamura Y, Ono H, Zhou X, Frohlich ED: Angiotensin type 1 receptor antagonism and ACE inhibition produce similar renoprotection in L-NAME/SHR rats. *Hypertension* 2001;**37**:1262–1267.

Zhou X, Frohlich ED: Functional and structural involvement of afferent and efferent glomerular arterioles in hypertension. *Am. J. Kidney Dis.* 2001;**37**:1092–1097.

Ono H, Ono Y, Takanohashi A, Matsuoha H, Frohlich ED: Apoptosis and glomerular injury after prolonged nitric oxide synthase inhibition in SHR. *Hypertension* 2001;**38**:1300–1306.

Zhou X, Ono H, Ono Y, Frohlich ED: N- and L-type calcium channel antagonistic improves glomerular dynamics, reverses severe nephrosclerosis and inhibits apoptosis and proliferation in an L-NAME/SHR model. *J. Hypertens.* 2002;**20**:993–1000.

Zhou X, Ono H, Ono Y, Frohlich ED: Aldosterone antagonism ameliorates proteinuria and nephrosclerosis independent of glomerular dynamics in L-NAME/SHR model. *Am. J. Nephrol.* 2004;**24**:242–249.

Zhou X, Matavelli LC, Ono H, Frohlich ED: Superiority of combination of thiazide with angiotensin-converting enzyme inhibitor or AT_1-receptor blocker over thiazide alone on renoprotection in L-NAME/SHR. *Am. J. Physiol.* 2005;**289**:F871–F879.

Zhou X, Frohlich ED: Analogy of cardiac and renal complications in essential hypertension and aged SHR or L-NAME/SHR. *Med. Chem.* 2007;**3**:61–65.

Matavelli LC, Zhou X, Varagic J, Susic D, Frohlich ED: Salt loading produces severe renal hemodynamic dysfunction independent of arterial pressure in spontaneously hypertensive rats. *Am. J. Physiol. Heart Circ. Physiol.* 2007;**292**:H814–H819.

Papers related to involvement of the kidney in hypertension

Hostetter TH, Olson JL, Rennke HG, Venkatachalam MA, Brenner BM: Hyperfiltration in remnant nephrons: a potentially adverse response to renal ablation. *Am. J. Physiol.* 1981;**241**:F85–F93.

Brenner BM, Meyer TW, Hostetter TH: Dietary protein intake and the progressive nature of kidney disease: the tale of hemodynamically mediated glomerular disease in the pathogenesis of progressive glomerular sclerosis in aging, renal ablation, and intrinsic renal disease. *N. Engl. J. Med.* 1982;**307**:652–659.

Brenner BM, Cooper ME, de Zeeuw D, Keane WF, Parving HH, *et al.*: Effects of losartan on renal and cardiovascular outcomes in patients with type 2 diabetes and nephropathy. *N. Engl. J. Med.* 2001;**345**:861–869.

US Renal Data Systems. 1995 Annual Data Report. National Institutes of Health, National Institute of Diabetes, Digestive and Kidney Diseases, III: incidence and causes of treated ESRD. *Am. J. Kidney Dis.* 1995;**26**:S39–50.

UKPDS Group. UK Prospective Diabetes Study 38: tight blood pressure control and risk of macrovascular and microvascular complications in type 2 diabetes. *BMJ* 1998; **317**:703–713.

The Seventh Report of the Joint National Committee on Prevention, Detection, Evaluation, and Treatment of High Blood Pressure (JNC-7). *JAMA* 2003;**289**:2560–2572,.

UKPDS Group: Efficacy of atenolol and captopril in reducing risk of macrovascular and microvascular complications in type 2 diabetes. UKPDA 39. *BMJ* 1998;**317**:713–720.

Frohlich ED: Arthur C. Corcoran Memorial Lecture: Influence of nitric oxide and angiotensin II on renal involvement in hypertension. *Hypertension* 1997;**29**:188–193.

Lewis EJ, Hunsickeer LG, Bain RP, Rohde RD: The effect of angiotensin converting-enzyme inhibition on diabetic nephropathy. The Collaborative Study Group. *N. Engl. J. Med.* 1993;**320**:1456–1462.

Sowers JR, Epstein M, Frohlich ED: Diabetes, hypertension and cardiovascular disease: An update. *Hypertension* 2001;**37**:1053–1059.

Hansson L, Lindholm LH, Niskanen L, Lanke J, Hedner T, Niklason A, et al: Effect of angiotensin-converting-enzyme inhibition compared with conventional therapy on cardiovascular morbidity and mortality in hypertension: the Captopril Prevention Project (CAPPP) randomized trial. *Lancet* 1999;**353**:611–616.

Sowers JR, Frohlich ED: Insulin and insulin resistance: Impact on blood pressure and cardiovascular disease. *Med. Clin. North Am.* 2004;**88**:63–82.

Parving HH, Lehnert H, Brochner-Mortensen J, Gomis R, Andersen S, Arner P: The effect of ibesartan on the development of diabetic nephropathy in patients with type 2 diabetes. *N. Engl. J. Med.* 2001; **345**:870–878.

Zhou X, Frohlich ED: Ageing, hypertension and the kidney: new data on an old problem. *Nephrology Dialysis Transplantation* 2003;**18:**1442–445.

Yusuf S, Sleight P, Pogue J, Bosch J, Davies R, Dagenais G: Effects of an angiotensin-converting-enzyme inhibitor, ramipril, on cardiovascular events in high-risk patients: the Heart Outcomes Prevention Evaluation Study Investigators. *N. Engl. Med.* 2000;**342**:145–153.

Zhou X, Frohlich ED: Differential effects of pharmacological interventions on renal injury in the experimental model of chronic nitric oxide inhibition. *Am J Nephrol.* 2005; 25:138–152.

Bakris Gl, Barnhill BW, Sadler R: Treatment of arterial hypertension in diabetic humans: importance of therapeutic selection. *Kidney Int.* 1992;**41**:912–919.

Frohlich ED: Target organ involvement in hypertension: A realistic promise of prevention and reversal. *Med. Clin. North Am.* 2004; **88**:209–221.

Mann JF, Gerstein HC, Pogue J, Bosch J, Yusuf S: Renal insufficiency as a predictor of cardiovascular outcomes and the impact of ramipril: the HOPE randomized trial. *Ann. Intern. Med.* 2001;**134**:629–636.

Matavelli LC, Zhou X, Frohlich ED: Hypertensive renal vascular disease andcardiovascular endpoints. *Curr. Opin. Cardiol.* 2006; **21**:305–309.

Yokoyama H, Tomonaga O, Hirayama M, Ishii A, Takeda M, Babazono T, et al: Predictors of the progression of diabetic nephropathy and the beneficial effect of angiotensin-converting enzyme inhibitors in NIDDM patients. *Diabetologia* 1997;**40**:405–411.

Bakris GL, Weir MR, DeQuattro V, McMahon FG: Effects of an ACE inhibitor/calcium antagonist combination on proteinuria in diabetic nephropathy. *Kidney Int.* 1998;**54**:1283–1289.

Zhou X, Frohlich ED: Physiologic evidence of renoprotection by antihypertensivetherapy. *Curr. Opin. Cardiol.* 2005;**20**:290–295.

Zhou X, Matavelli LC, Frohlich ED: Uric acid: its relationship to renalhemodynamics and the renal renin-angiotensin system. *Curr. Hypertens. Rep.* 2006;**8**:120–124.

Berl T, Hunsicker LG, Lewis JB, Pfeffer MA, Porush JG, Rouleau JL, et al:Cardiovascular outcomes in the Irbesartan Diabetic Nephropathy Trial of patients with type 2 diabetes and overt nephropathy. *An.n Intern. Med.* 2003;**138**:542–549.

Thomas MC, Cooper ME, Shahinfar S, Brenner BM: Dialysis delayed is deathprevented: a clinical perspective on the RENAAL study. *Kidney Int.* 2003; **63**:1577–1579.

Manjunath G, Tighiouart H, Coresh J, Macleod B, Salem DN, Griffith JL, et.al: Level of kidney function as a risk factor for cardiovascular outcomes in the elderly. *Kidney Int.* 2003; **63**:1121–1129.

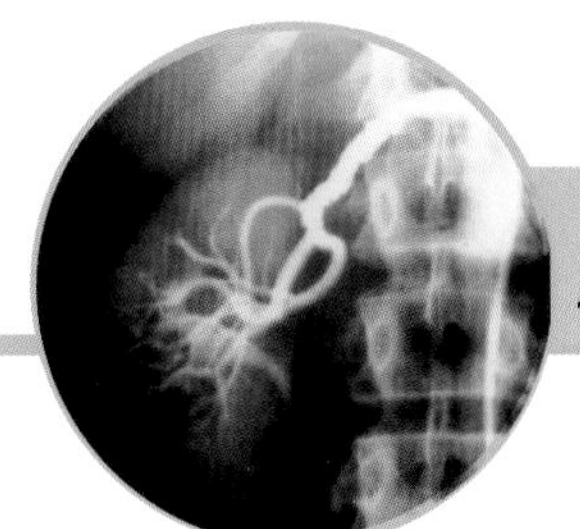

Chapter 7

Renal arterial disease

Introduction

Several general considerations are worth stating before considering the clinical problem of hypertension resulting from (or exacerbated by) occlusive renal arterial disease.

First, occlusive renal arterial lesions occur in normotensive as well as hypertensive individuals, especially if these patients have other occlusive atherosclerotic lesions elsewhere in the circulation. Thus, atherosclerotic renal arterial lesions are not infrequently observed in normotensive patients undergoing renal arteriography for a comprehensive assessment of atherosclerotic disease of other organs. This concept is worth considering at this point since renal arteriography is frequently obtained as a more comprehensive study associated with coronary and peripheral arteriography.

Second, renal arterial disease associated with elevated arterial pressure (i.e. renovascular hypertension) is often said to be a rare secondary cause of systemic arterial hypertension and yet it occurs in 3–5% of all patients with hypertension. Using a conservative estimate of the current prevalence of hypertension in the USA, upwards of 2.5 million patients with hypertension may have renal arterial disease. And, of course, the disease occurs with increasing frequency in elderly patients since atherosclerotic lesions and hypertensive blood pressure levels are more frequent in this age group.

Third, renal arterial disease may complicate the course of essential hypertension, especially in those older people whose blood pressure has become more difficult to control (*Table 7.1*).

Pathophysiology

As suggested above, since both normotensive and hypertensive patients may have renal arterial lesions, they become clinically significant only when the lesions compromise renal and intrarenal haemodynamics sufficiently to stimulate the renopressor system or to adversely affect renal parenchymal function. When renal haemodynamics is sufficiently compromised, release of renin from the juxtaglomerular apparatus is increased and this, in turn, generates the production of angiotensin II. The increased angiotensin II generated raises arterial pressure through two

Table 7.1 Clinical cues suggesting renovascular hypertension

- Severe hypertension in a young child, young adult or an adult older than 50 years
- Sudden development of or worsening of pre-existing hypertension at any age
- Systolic/diastolic, upper abdominal or flank bruits
- Hypertension associated with unexplained impairment of renal function (suggesting bilateral disease)
- Impaired renal function in response to an ACE inhibitor, suggesting bilateral disease
- Sudden worsening of renal function in a hypertensive patient
- Elevation of blood pressure refractory to the appropriate three-drug regimen
- Development of accelerated or malignant hypertension
- Unilateral small kidney discovered by any study
- Extensive occlusive atherosclerotic disease in the coronary, cerebral or other circulations

mechanisms: (1) arteriolar constriction, which increases total peripheral resistance; and (2) secondarily by promoting aldosterone release from the adrenal cortex, leading to the specific metabolic changes of secondary hyperaldosteronism manifested primarily by hypokalaemic alkalosis. This is established by demonstrating increased plasma renin activity (PRA), increased circulating aldosterone concentration and urinary secretion, and sodium and water retention.

In our experience, if the renin concentration in blood sampled from the renal veins is higher in the affected kidney than in the unaffected kidney by a factor of 1.6 or more, then this is strongly suggestive of a unilateral lesion. However, evaluation of bilateral renal arterial disease is less clear-cut. In addition, one must bear in mind that there often are multiple renal arteries and veins or there may be multiple or bilateral lesions. For this reason, additional markers associated with renal arterial lesions are actively being sought. Factors under active study in our institution include the elevation of brain natriuretic peptide (BNP), angiotensinogen and other factors.

Diagnosis

Clearly, the patient's clinical history is extremely valuable, since renal involvement is the most common secondary form of hypertension (excluding over-the-counter and street drugs). A number of screening laboratory tests have been made available for the diagnosis of significant renal arterial disease, each with varying sensitivity and specificity. However, the 'gold standard' for the clinical diagnosis (in our opinion) resides with careful selective renal arteriography since it confirms the presence of disease and the extent of renal arterial involvement, and provides an excellent means of assessing anatomy and haemodynamic function and natural history.

The size of the kidneys also provides an excellent index of the significance of the lesions. A smaller kidney suggests significant occlusive disease, although unilateral renal atrophy should always be considered. In this regard, the left kidney is normally 0.5 cm longer than the right; thus, a 1.0–1.5 cm difference in the length of the kidneys should arouse suspicion. The delayed appearance of radiographic contrast material on intravenous urography with hyperconcentration and delay of disappearance should also provoke some suspicion; however, intravenous urography is less frequently used today.

Radioactive renography may also be helpful, with a delayed appearance and disappearance of the tagged radionuclide being of some value although this study is, at best, a 'screening test'. However, preoperative and postoperative isotopic renography (with renal flow and scan) may be useful procedures in order to help evaluation of postoperative increased arterial pressure. Renographic studies before and after administration of a rapidly acting ACE inhibitor (i.e. captopril) associated with measurements of PRA may suggest a significant lesion, but again this approach is less useful nowadays. Finally, measurement of PRA (indexed to daily sodium intake) may also be of value but may be fraught with pitfalls and can be affected by diet and concurrent therapy. In summary, if one is seriously considering renal arterial disease, we believe that visualization of the renal arteries is in order and, overall, this is, in our opinion, probably the most cost-effective study.

Types of arterial lesions

The pathological nature of renal arterial lesions has an important bearing on the natural history of the disease. Identification of the renal arterial lesion arteriographically should be of great value in defining the pathological type of the lesion.

If the renal arterial disease is unilateral, treating the patient with an ACE inhibitor will inhibit the amount of angiotensin II that will be generated and, therefore, will reduce the level of the arterial pressure. However, if the patient has bilateral occlusive disease of the renal arteries, both kidneys will become ischaemic and will release increased amounts of renin. As a result, renal parenchymal function may become impaired. Arterial lesions may broadly be considered to be either atherosclerotic or non-atherosclerotic (or fibrosing); and the latter lesions are variable (*Table 7.2*).

In evaluating the patient with a renal arterial lesion, consideration should be given to several potential complications (*Table 7.3*).

In this discussion, we shall rely greatly on the older techniques of aortography as well as selective renal arteriography as earlier studies from the Cleveland Clinic employing careful arteriographic, pathological and clinical correlations provided much important information on the natural history of the disease produced by these lesions (in

Table 7.2 Various types of renal arterial disease and hypertension

Atherosclerotic

Non-atherosclerotic (fibrosing)

1. Intimal fibroplasia
2. Medial (or perimedial) fibroplasia
3. Subadventitial fibroplasia
4. Fibromuscular hyperplasia

Embolic

1. Tumour
2. Suture
3. Fibrosis (drugs, radiation)

particular, the fibrosing lesions). Hence, this discussion is unique since clinical studies and treatment today do not usually include removal of renal arterial segments to correlate with the arteriographic and clinical pictures.

Atherosclerotic lesions

Patients with these lesions may present with specific clinical features (*Table 7.4*). These lesions are usually located at the orifice or the proximal one-third of the main renal artery. The selective arteriogram usually demonstrates eccentricity of the occlusive lesion (**7.1**) or it may appear as post-stenotic dilatation, having a 'boggy' or balloon-like appearance (**7.2**).

Atherosclerotic lesions are more common in men aged 45 years or older. If the patient is older, the lesions may be bilateral and the atherosclerosis may be more diffuse, even involving the aorta and other organs. Pathologically, the lesions may be intimal in location (**7.3**) and may be complicated by dissection (**7.4**). Because of this potential, before surgical repair is considered, the patient should be evaluated fully for disease involving the coronary, carotid, splanchnic and peripheral arteries as well as the aorta. Awareness of these possibilities should stimulate consideration of the feasibility of angioplasty or, more frequently, intravascular stent placement. If either type of repair is considered, one should take into consideration not only the occlusive lesion, but the purpose of the operative procedure: cure of the hypertensive disease; improved control of arterial pressure (even if drug therapy will still be necessary); preservation of renal function; or management of the secondary problems of the arterial disease (e.g. dissection, rupture, repair of bleeding, thrombosis associated with severe pain and/or dissection). In most situations, today, stent placement is preferable.

Table 7.3 Complications resulting from renal arterial disease

1. Thrombosis
2. Aneurysmal formation
3. Dissection
4. Haemorrhage
5. Metabolic

Table 7.4 Clinical features in patients with atherosclerotic lesions

- Older patients
- Men (under 50 years)
- Hyperlipidaemias
- Evaluate other major arteries
- Assess renal function

Non-atherosclerotic (fibrosing) lesions

Fibrosing lesions of the renal artery are associated with different natural histories; and each type of lesion seems to have a different natural history. Fortunately, fibrosing lesions have very different radiographic appearances, depending upon the involved layer(s) of the renal arterial wall. As indicated above, due credit for our understanding of these lesions must be given to the radiologists, pathologists, surgeons and clinicians at the Cleveland and Mayo Clinics who, in the 1960s and 1970s, elucidated the fascinating and important correlations between their arteriographic, pathological and clinical characteristics. At that time, it was their practice to resect the entire arterial lesion and then reconstitute the continuity of the artery. Thus, they were able to correlate the pathological alterations with their radiographic appearance and the clinical history of the patients involved.

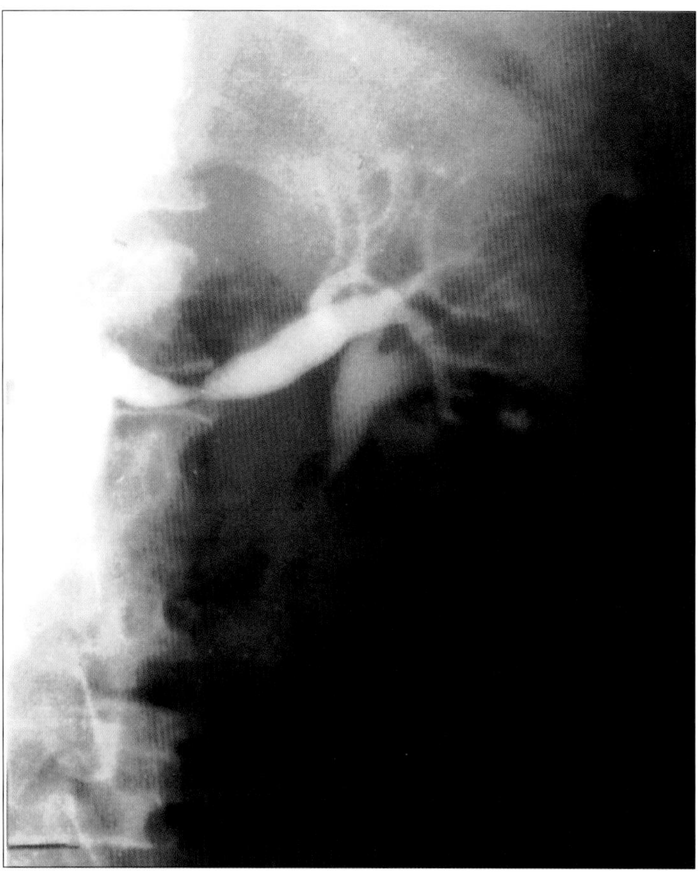

7.1 Atherosclerotic left renal arterial lesion demonstrating its eccentricity in location.

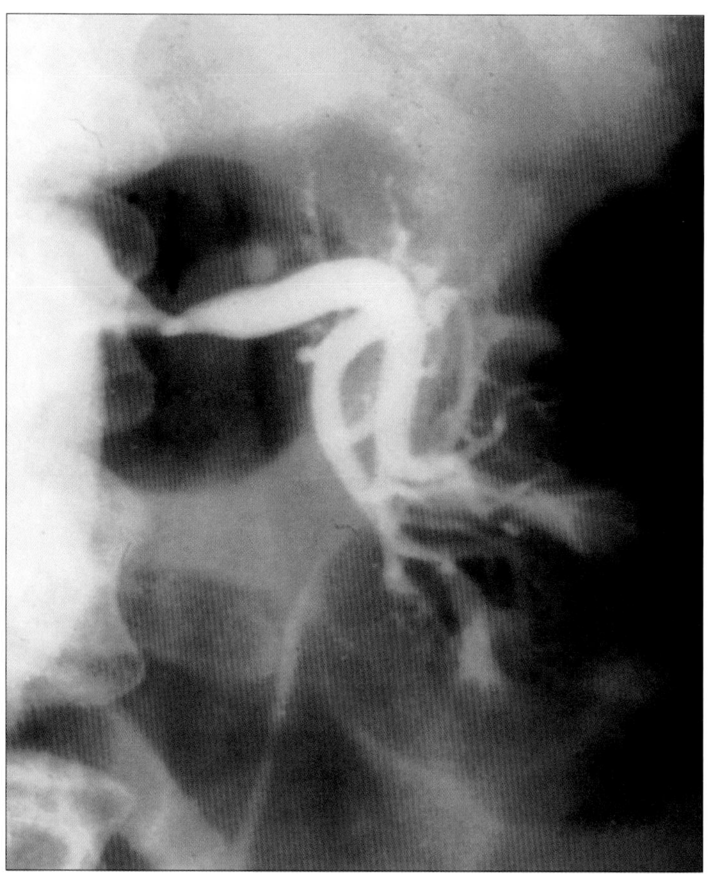

7.2 Atherosclerotic left renal arterial lesion demonstrating a tight stenosis with post-stenotic dilation and 'bogginess' or a balloon-type appearance.

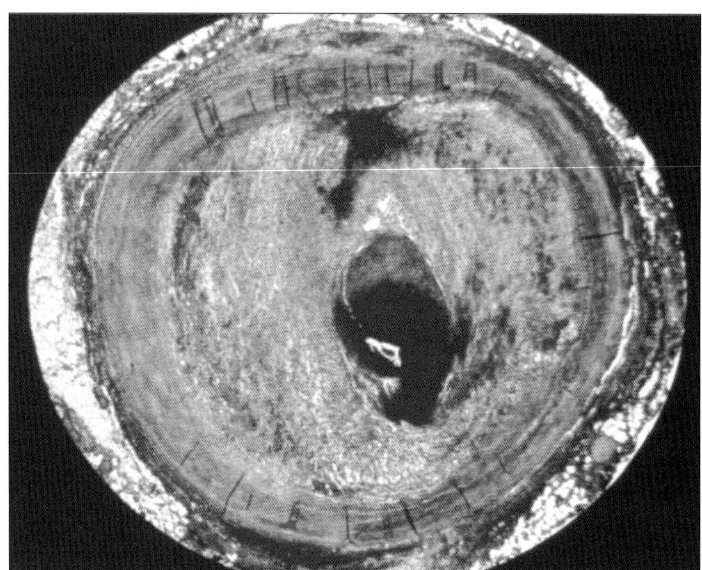

7.3 Cross-sectional micrograph of the left renal artery showing almost total vascular occlusion from intimal obliteration due to atherosclerosis.

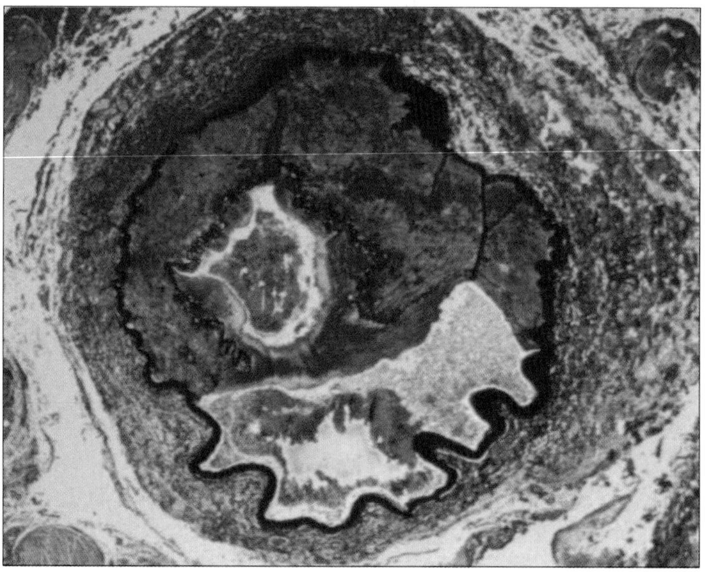

7.4 Cross-sectional micrograph of the right renal artery demonstrating almost total luminal occlusion with evidence of dissection due to atherosclerosis.

Medial fibroplasia

Perhaps the most common of the fibrosing lesions is *medial* (or *perimedial*) *fibroplasia*. This abnormality is not infrequently bilateral, occurs more commonly in younger women and, on arteriography, is not severely stenosing and has the classical appearance of the so-called 'string of beads' lesion (**7.5**). This lesion appears as multifocal sequential areas of fibrosis within the media of the arterial wall that do not disrupt the external limiting membrane of the media (**7.6** and **7.7**).

The disease disrupts the internal elastic membrane while the external elastic membrane remains intact, thereby giving the classical arteriographic appearance of a 'string of beads'. The disease, fortunately, progresses slowly and may be rarely complicated by dissection or rupture of the aneurysmal dilatations. For this reason, the patient may be followed over a longer time period while receiving pharmacotherapeutic agents unless blood pressure and renal function control are difficult. Hence, we believe that this lesion can be managed with an anti-hypertensive agent that can be selected to inhibit the renin–angiotensin system [e.g. ACE inhibitors or angiotensin II (type 1) receptor antagonists]. It is important, however, to point out that these agents should not be prescribed if the renal arterial disease is bilateral or in a patient with unilateral renal arterial disease in a solitary kidney (see discussion above). Under such circumstances, we have found that a calcium antagonist (e.g. diltiazem, verapamil) may be very useful.

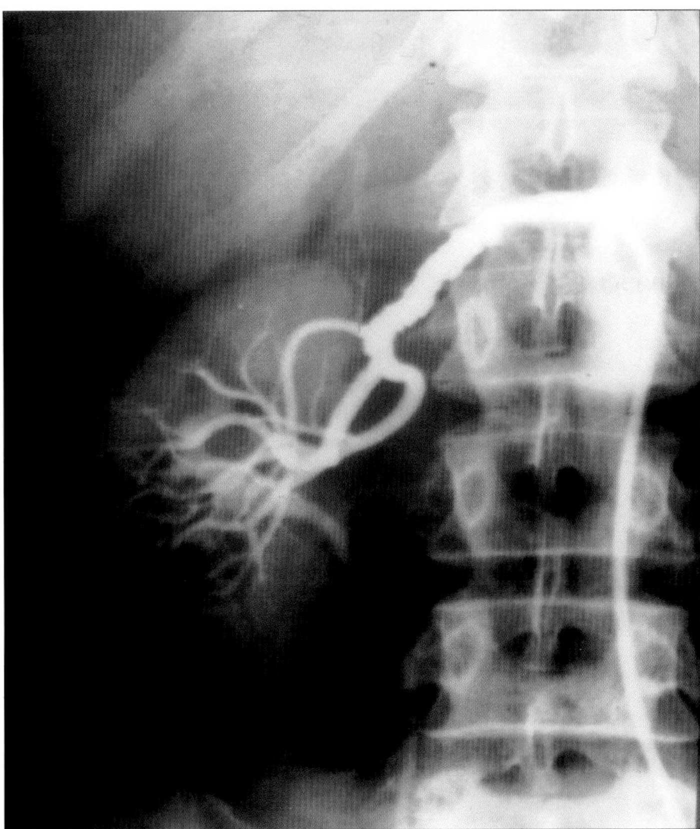

7.5 The classical 'string of beads' radiographic appearance in this right renal artery with medial fibroplasia.

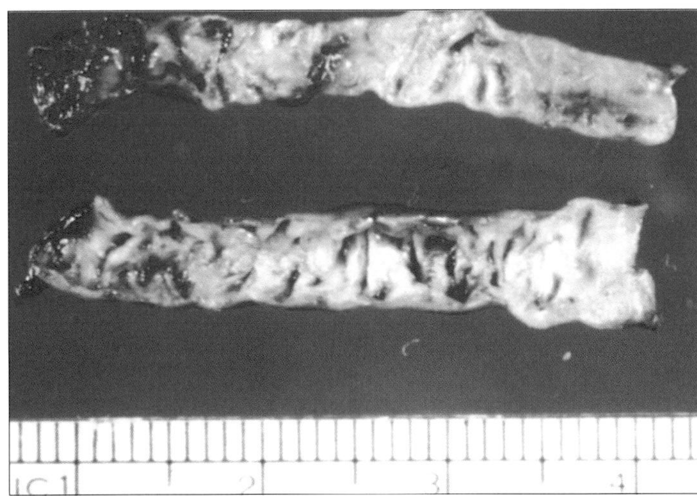

7.6 Gross anatomical appearance of a longitudinal cut of a main renal artery with medial fibroplasia.

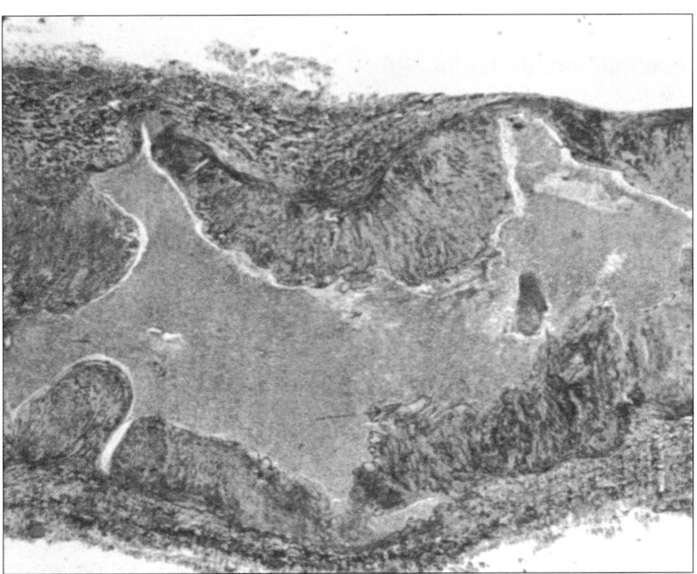

7.7 Low-magnification view of a main renal artery with medial fibroplasia demonstrating the intact external elastic membrane thereby accounting for the infrequency of dissection or progression of the lesion.

The remaining renal arterial lesions are fibrosing pathologically, but they may be more severely stenosing. In contrast to the intramural location of medial fibroplastic disease are the fibroplastic lesions of intimal fibroplasia, subadventitial fibroplasia and the mixed lesion of fibromuscular hyperplasia.

Intimal fibroplasia

This lesion is manifested by the proliferation of fibrous disease in the intimal layer of the arterial wall that produces a smooth, generally more symmetric and highly stenosing lesion. The lesion is more severely stenosing, not usually involving the main renal artery at its orifice, and may be complicated by occlusion, thrombosis, dissection or rupture. It seems to occur with equal frequency in men and women. Severely stenotic lesions of intimal fibroplasia of renal arteries that are characteristically non-orificial and may be complicated by thrombosis, occlusion or dissection are shown in **7.8–7.10.**

Micrographs of renal arteries demonstrating intimal fibroplasia are shown in **7.11** and **7.12**.

Intimal fibroplasia lesions, like the atherosclerotic lesions, may occur in the proximal third of the renal artery, although they may also occur more distally and are characterized by a circumferential proliferation of fibrous tissue within the intimal layer of the vessel wall. On arteriography, the lesion may have a more symmetrical stenotic appearance that produces a more severe physiological impairment of vascular haemodynamics. The lesions may occur in children as well as in adults, and there does not seem to be a gender preference. The lesion of intimal fibroplasia severely restricts the arterial lumen, and is complicated by severely elevated arterial pressures and arterial complications including dissection, rupture with haemorrhage and thrombosis; collateralization of the kidney may also occur (**7.8–7.12**).

Subadventitial fibroplasia

This fibrosing disease produces a severely stenosing lesion with the radiological appearance of aneurysms that are less confluent than those of medial fibroplasia. The aneurysmal dissection reflects disruption of the external limiting membrane and there may be a characteristic collateral flow

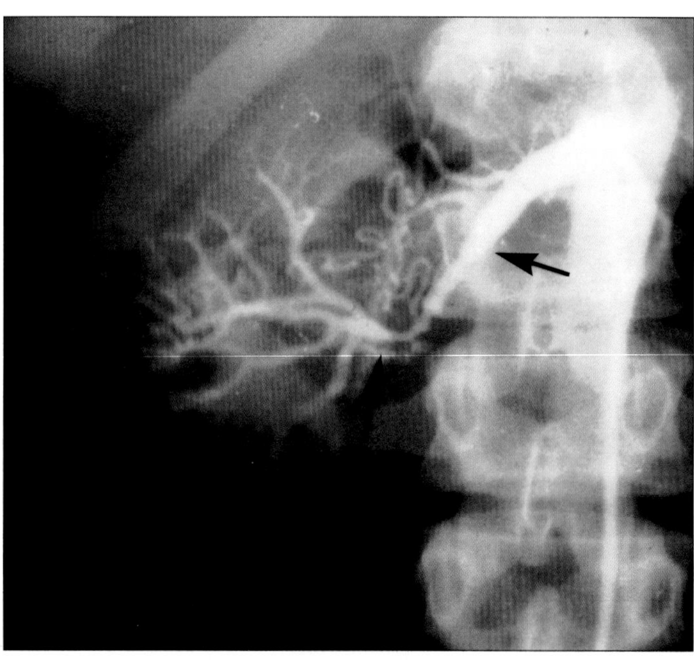

7.8 Intimal fibroplasia of the right main renal artery and a primary (lower) branch. Note the aneurysmal dilatations of the lesions. Most notable is the development of collateral vascularity emanating from the renal artery distally into the renal parenchyma.

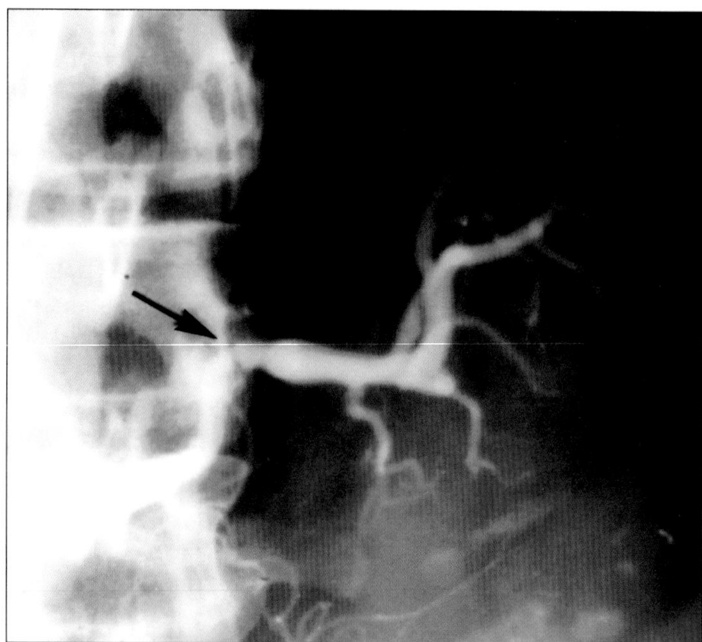

7.9 Intimal fibroplasia of the initial (post-ostial) part of the left renal artery with involvement of the main renal artery distally. Note also the collateralization of vessels into the parenchyma of the kidney.

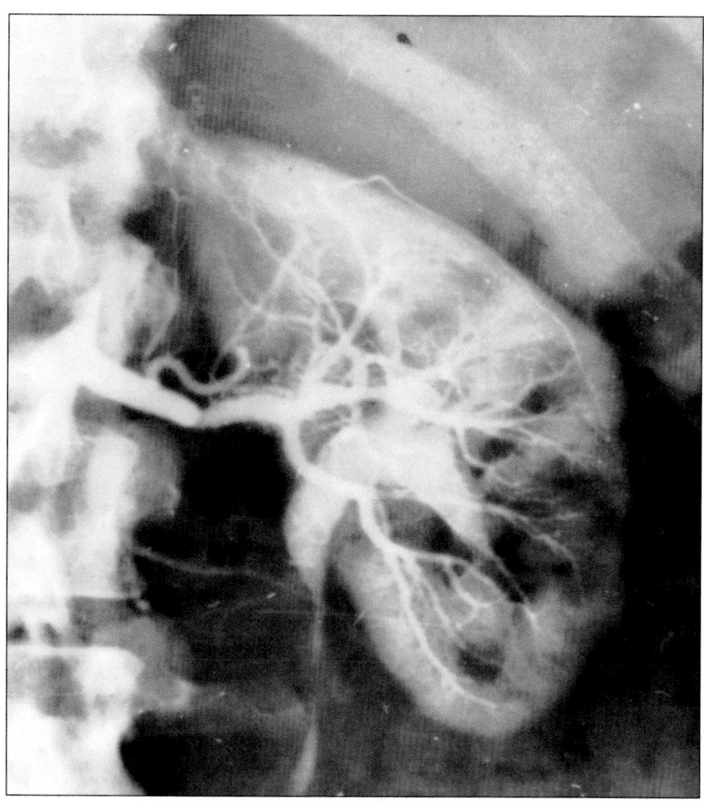

7.10 Intimal fibroplasia of the left renal artery with more distal involvement of that vessel. Note the collateralization of vessels throughout the upper half of the kidney distally to the renal capsule.

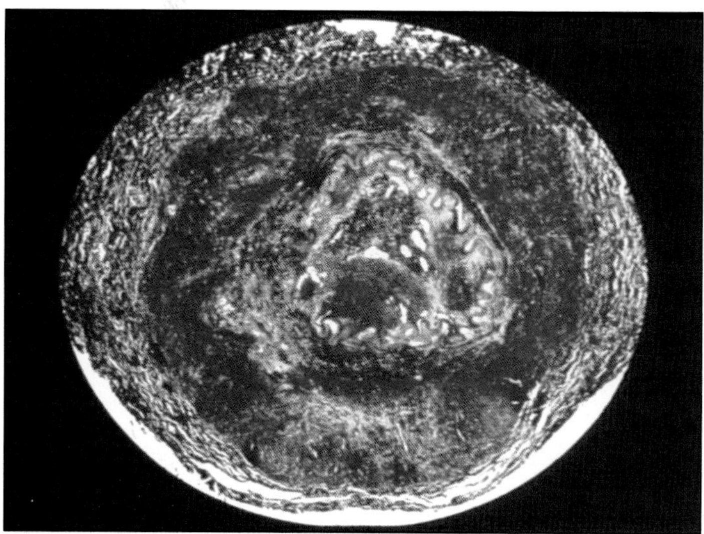

7.11 Cross-section of a severely stenosed renal arterial lesion (depicted in **7.10** arteriogram) produced by intimal fibroplasia. Fibrous tissue demonstrated by Masson stain.

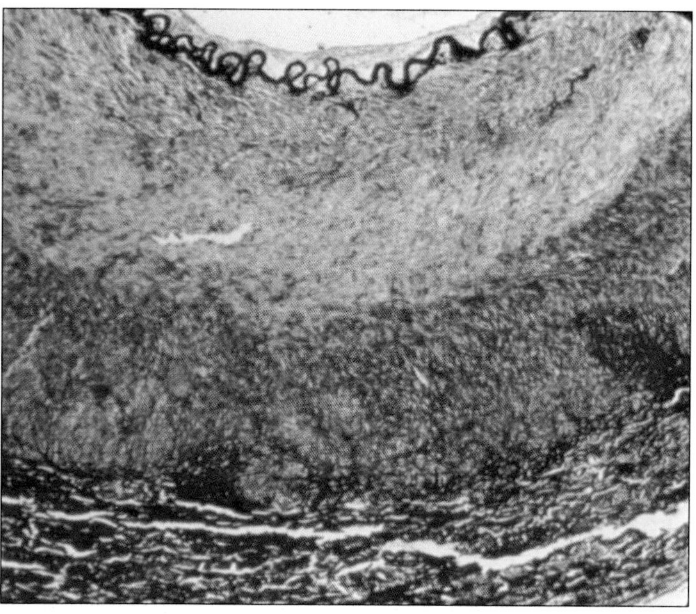

7.12 Section of artery with markedly thickened intima demonstrating intimal fibroplasia. The lumen of the artery is above with an intact internal elastic lamina membrane.

surrounding the artery and the upper part of the kidney, indicating considerable renal ischaemia (**7.13** and **7.14**).

Microscopically, the lesions are characteristically located in the subadventitia with severe fibrosis. The lesions of subadventitial fibroplasia appear arteriographically as severe stenosis, with fibrous tissue frequently invading the external elastic membrane to involve the subadventitial area of the arterial wall. The disease can cause a variety of luminal irregularities, and marked development of collateral vessels is often seen on the arteriogram. These lesions are frequently complicated by involvement of both kidneys; and the disease may be associated with dissection and haemorrhage. Although pharmacological therapy may frequently be useful, the clinician should consider early and periodic surgical consultation with repeated selective arteriographic studies if surgical or invasive angioplastic treatment is not pursued.

Fibromuscular hyperplasia

In contrast to the fibrosing lesions described above, fibromuscular hyperplasia (a term that is frequently wrongly used) is the least frequent of the fibrosing lesions and is manifested histologically by both fibrous and muscular disease of the arterial wall (**7.16** and **7.17**). The lesions are also severely stenosing (**7.18**) and may be manifested by gross aneurysmal dilatations even into the more distal areas of the artery. Microscopically, the arterial wall layers are involved by fibrosis with smooth muscle cells interspersed. The disease may occur bilaterally and is frequently associated with collateralization and complicated by thrombosis, dissection and haemorrhage.

Conclusion

Thus, renal arterial disease and hypertension is a very complex disease physiologically, anatomically, structurally, pathologically and clinically. However, with careful evaluation clinically, arteriographically and therapeutically the patients can be managed effectively and successfully.

Suggested reading

The reader is referred to the next chapter, Concluding remarks, for suggested reading for this chapter.

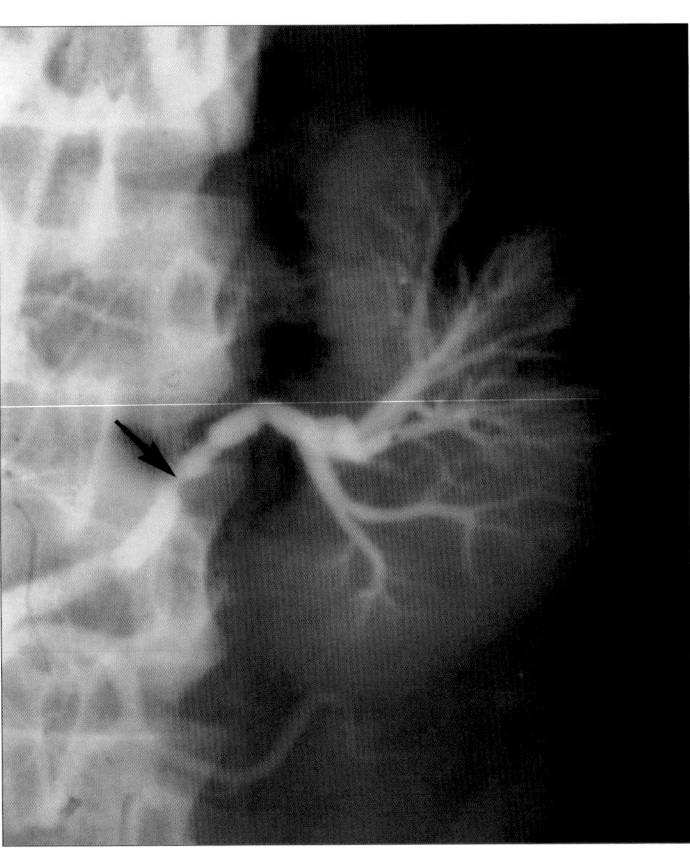

7.13 Severely stenosing renal arterial lesion of subadventitial fibroplasia.

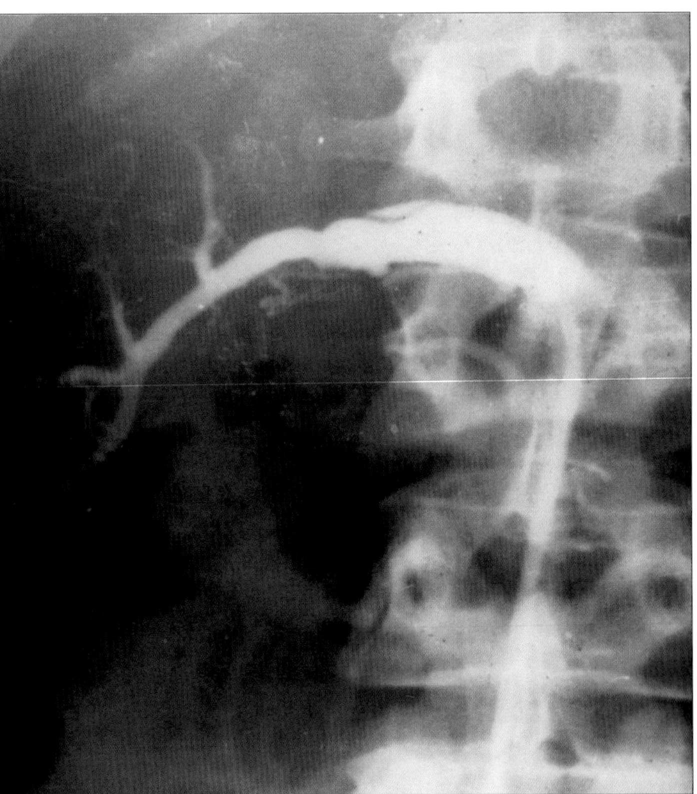

7.14 Severely stenosing renal arterial lesion of subadventitial fibroplasia manifested by collateralization.

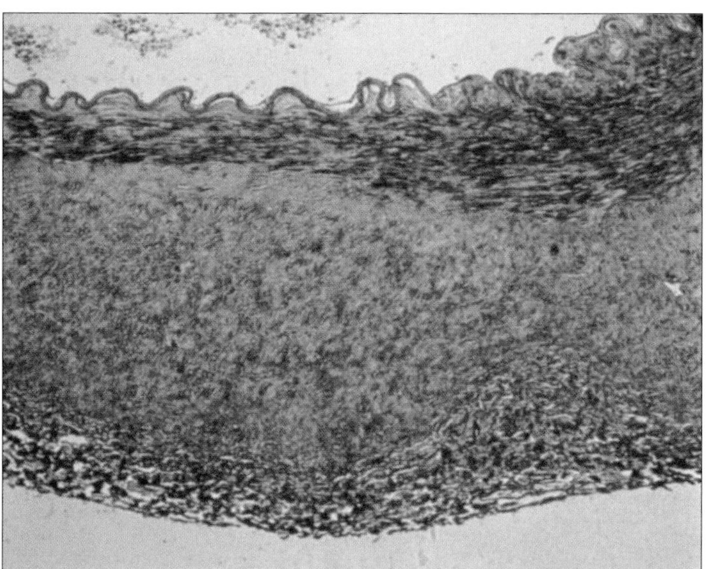

7.15 Microscopic section of the wall from the vessel depicted in Fig. 7.13. Note the wide subadventitial area with fibrosis accounting for the severe restriction of flow.

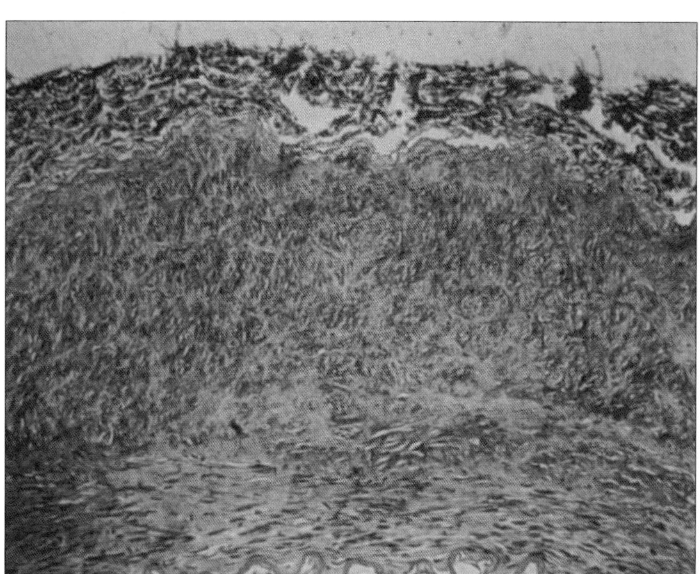

7.16 Microscopic section of renal arterial wall of the artery depicting the marked fibromuscular infiltration of the media and the disruption of the external limiting membrane.

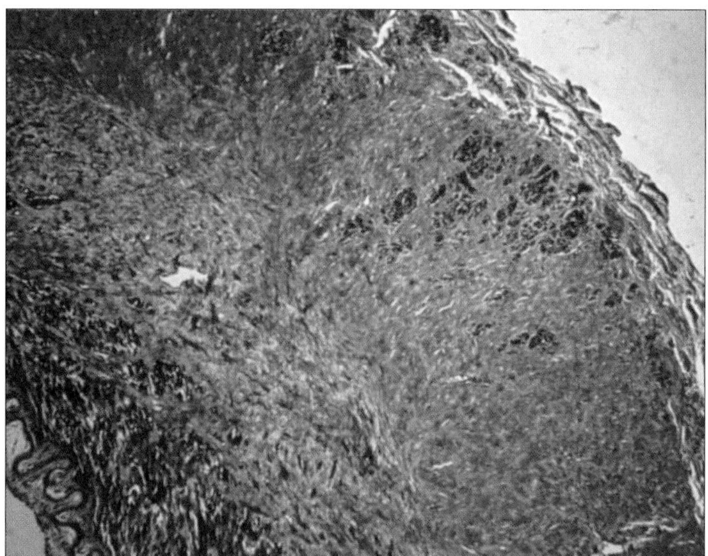

7.17 Another microscopic section of the above vessel wall stained to present the dramatic widening of the vessel media, its infiltration by smooth muscle cells (in red) as well as the fibrosis (in blue).

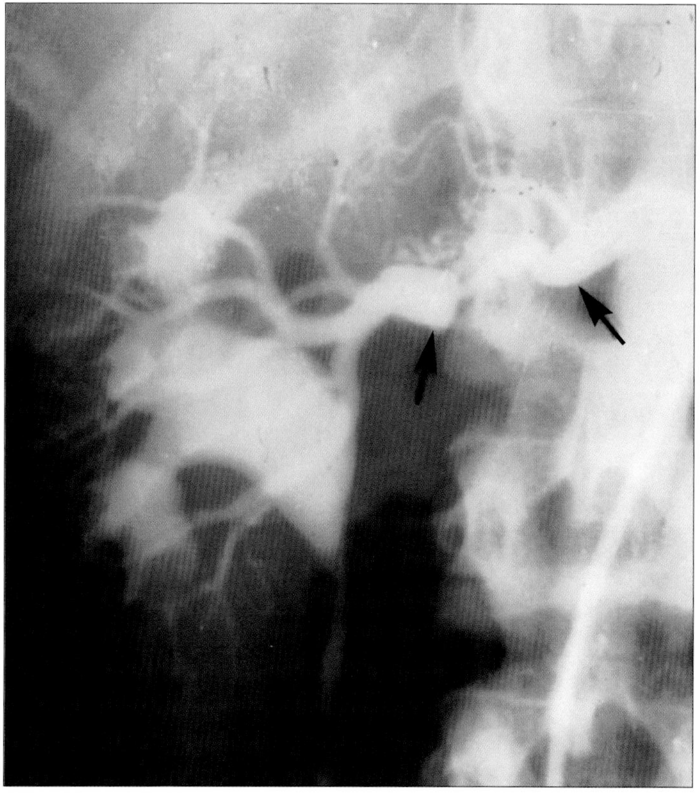

7.18 Severely stenosing lesions of fibromuscular hyperplasia demonstrating collateral vascalarity, aneurysmal formation with post-stenotic dilatation of the affected right renal artery.

Chapter 8

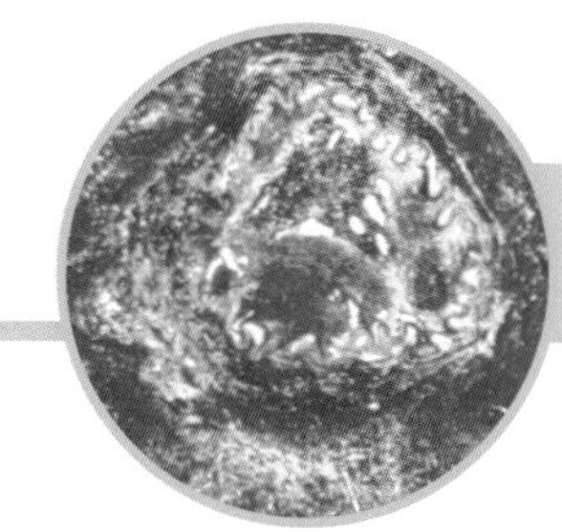

Concluding comments

As stated in our Preface and Introduction, one of the prime intentions in publishing this atlas was to put together, in one volume, a personal overview of current knowledge concerning the pathophysiology, clinical and diagnostic evaluation and the clinical treatment of the patient with essential hypertension.

Part of the diagnostic evaluation of the patient with hypertension is consideration of the role of renal arterial disease. However, there is little in the current literature about the pathological, radiographic and clinical natural history correlations of specific renal arterial lesions. Much of this information resides in the literature of the early 1960s written by my dear friends and colleagues at the Cleveland Clinic, Harriet P. Dustan, MD, and Thomas F. Meaney, MD, of the Research Division and Department of Radiology. Their work was importantly supported by the remarkable surgical repair of renal arterial lesions by Eugene Poutasse, MD, and by the pathological studies of these lesions by Lawrence J. McCormack of the Departments of Urology and Pathology, respectively. In contrast to the present state of the art, whereby renal arterial lesions are treated by placement of stents, direct intravascular arterial dilatation or surgically, these renal arterial lesions were carefully excised and then end-to-end arterial reanastomosis was used to reinstate continuity of blood flow to the affected kidney. The patients were followed carefully by periodic radiographic examinations prior to and following the renal arterial surgery, thereby providing a unique presentation of the natural history of renal arterial disease.

Fortunately, Doctor Dustan provided me with some of her slide library of these lesions before her death and, in homage to these outstanding clinicians and investigators, I have included their experiences in this atlas and acknowledge their landmark contributions. These experiences should be of great value to those clinicians interested in the pathophysiology and natural history of hypertensive renal arterial disease. I doubt whether any similar documents are available to the practising physician today. And, on a much more personal note, one might be interested in how and why these physicians were able to perform these procedures at a time when Mason F. Sones, MD, of the Clinic's Department of Cardiology had only recently introduced his technique of intra-arterial catheterization and arteriography of the coronary arteries. At that time Mason Sones was tremendously preoccupied with the number of patients referred to him for his new procedure of direct coronary artery catheterization and angiography. Hence, at a meeting organized by Harriet Dustan, he agreed to catheterize arteries above the diaphragm (with the exception of the arterial supply to the brain), and Tom Meaney introduced the technique of direct renal arterial catheterization for the diagnosis of renal arterial disease. At the time, renal arteriography was achieved by aortograms, a much inferior technique to visualize the arterial supply to the kidney.

I remember well that each of these physicians at the Cleveland Clinic was concerned with the then-current and still-used single term for the various fibrosing lesions of the renal arteries. We don't even refer to the term 'fibromuscular hyperplasia' since this is a term for a more specific fibrosing lesion. In deference to their remarkable contributions, here we follow the terminology they originally suggested.

On a different line of thinking, rather than discuss and present at length the various biological and pathological mechanisms associated with arterial pressure elevation, we have presented these concepts only more generally in order to preserve the purpose of presenting primarily clinical and pathophysiological information. As our knowledge of the biological and pathophysiological mechanisms subserving the maintenance, elevation or reduction of arterial pressure continues to increase exponentially each year, a detailed discussion of this may detract from our overall purpose of this atlas. Rather, therefore, we chose to discuss those mechanisms which merit discussion clinically and to emphasize their effects on the target organ involvement in essential hypertension.

As suggested in our discussions, it has been clearly demonstrated (even in the very earliest of the double-blinded multicentre trials) that arterial pressure reduction resulting from antihypertensive therapy reduces the risk of the morbidity and mortality associated with strokes. As has been pointed out from the earliest physiological and clinical literature, circulation to the brain is primarily maintained by an autoregulatory pressure mechanism. Consequently, these early clinical studies were terminated when the number of strokes experienced in the placebo-treated groups significantly exceeded the number occurring in the actively treated groups. There ensued much speculation that the other target organ end-points were affected adversely by diuretic therapy. However, more recent trials, employing lower doses of diuretics, resulting in significantly improved coronary heart disease outcomes, reaching values that are almost identical to the predictions made by the triallists' earliest meta-analysis. It should not be inferred that pressure reduction and control are less important for other target organs (heart, vessels, and kidneys); however, it is clear that other pressure mechanisms are clearly critical in the structural and functional involvement of the heart, vessels, and kidneys in hypertension. Indeed, we have presented detailed evidence that these mechanisms are common to the impairment blood flow, arteriolar constriction, fibrosis of the extracellular matrix and perivascularly, apoptosis and, perhaps, the inflammatory responses of these organs. Consideration of those mechanisms and their inhibition pharmacologically is the emphasis of much of this atlas. The experimental and clinical experience underlying our research over the past five decades therefore forms the substance of these chapters of the atlas.

Consequently, we express our deepest appreciation to the patients who have agreed to participate in the various investigations which provide our diagrammatic and pictorial presentations. In addition, we also express our appreciation to those institutions that have provided the ambiance and support necessary for us to conduct and report our investigative experiences. What a thrill it is to have begun these experiences at a time when effective therapy was not yet available and now to be able to control, prevent and (we believe) reverse the effects of this disease. Yet much remains to be done, and to this end we are committed.

Suggested reading

McCormack LJ, Poutassse EF, Meaney TF, Noto TJ Jr, Dustan HP: A pathologic-arteriographic correlation of renal arterial disease. *Am. Heart J.* 1966;**72**:188–198.

McCormack LJ, Noto TJ Jr, Meaney TF, Poutasse EF, Dustan HP: Subadvential fibroplasias of the renal artery, a disease of young women. *Am. Heart J.* 1967;**73**:602–614.

Meaney TF, Dustan HP, McCormack LJ: Natural history of renal arterial disease. *Radiology* 196891:881–887.

Dustan HP: Physiologic consequences of renal arterial stenosis. *N. Engl. J. Med.* 1969;**281**:1348–1354.

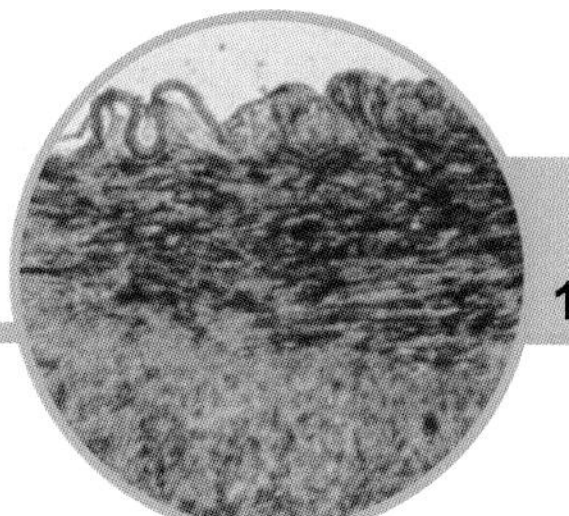

Epilogue

Epilogue

At the outset of this book, we expressed our thinking about this undertaking. We indicated our intention to convey the magnitude of the hypertension problem to primary care physicians – family doctors, general internists, cardiologists, nephrologists endocrinologists, obstetricians – and all who are interested in understanding their patients' diseases. Hypertension is a vast problem, afflicting over 1.2 billion people worldwide. The great majority of these potential patients have a disease that can be easily evaluated and treated without the need for hospitalization. What is further required, however, is a thorough understanding of the underlying pathophysiology of the disease and its complications. Two things are needed to accomplish this: a comprehension of some of the fundamental mechanisms that account for the maintenance of a normal blood pressure and a thirst to expand that knowledge as new information is continuingly being imparted. With such a fundamental and clinical background for this subject, it is then necessary to know how to evaluate expeditiously, and as inexpensively as possible, the patient for target organ involvement, complications, comorbid diseases and additional 'risk factors'. Having thus been imbued with an understanding of the patient and his or her disease, it is then necessary to understand the large number of available modes of therapy so that the underlying mechanisms of disease can be effectively counteracted by agents that can modify the natural history of that affliction. We have attempted to accomplish the foregoing with a special effort to focus on the two systems that are readily approached in the office practice setting; and these are the cardiovascular and renal systems. To this end, we hope that our goals have been accomplished and we humbly hope that readers have benefited from the personal and experimental lines of thinking of two other physicians whose experience in these areas and their patients have been the source of stimulation and satisfaction over these years.

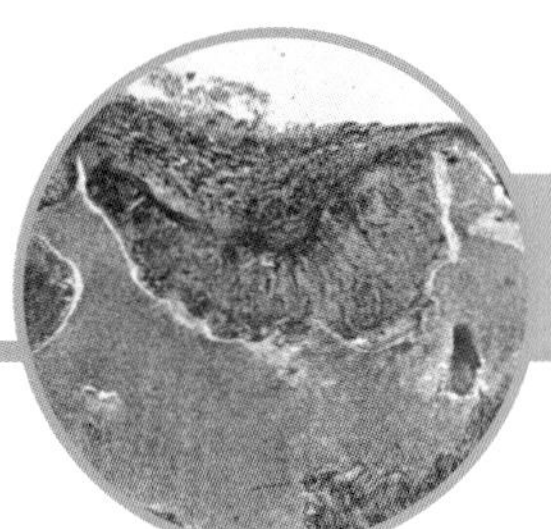

Index